SYNOPSIS IN THE MANAGEMENT OF URINARY INCONTINENCE

Edited by **Ammar Alhasso**
and **Holly Bekarma**

Synopsis in the Management of Urinary Incontinence
http://dx.doi.org/10.5772/62557
Edited by Ammar Alhasso and Holly Bekarma

Contributors

Mahmut Surmeli, Özlem Çinar Özdemir, Blanca Madurga Patuel, Candelaria Lafuente Molinero, Jose Luis Alvarez-Ossorio, Rodrigo Garcia-Baquero, M Hammad Ather, Raheela Mohsin Rizvi, Funda Gungor Ugurlucan, Xin-Yao Zhou, Ri Chang, Chun-Lan Jin, Ran Pang

Published by InTech

Janeza Trdine 9, 51000 Rijeka, Croatia

Publishing Process Manager Iva Lipovic
Technical Editor SPi Global
Cover InTech Design team

First published February, 2017
Printed in Croatia

Additional hard copies can be obtained from orders@intechopen.com

Synopsis in the Management of Urinary Incontinence, Edited by Ammar Alhasso and Holly Bekarma
p. cm.
Print ISBN 978-953-51-2931-8
Online ISBN 978-953-51-2932-5

For EU product safety concerns:
IN TECH d.o.o., Prolaz Marije Krucifikse Kozulić 3, 51000 Rijeka, Croatia,
info@intechopen.com or visit our website at intechopen.com.

Meet the editors

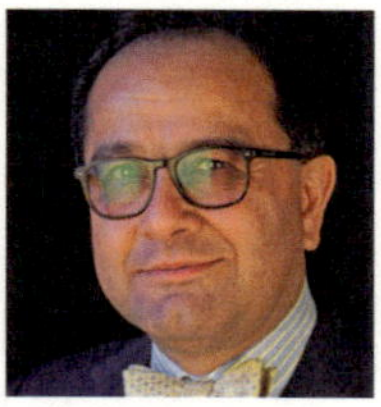

Ammar Alhasso is a consultant urological surgeon and lead in reconstructive urology, female urology and urodynamics at the University of Edinburgh Teaching Hospitals. He was a research fellow at Imperial College School of Medicine, University of London studying bladder cancer and obtained a Master degree in Surgical Sciences in 2000. He is also a reviewer for the Cochrane Collaboration/Incontinence Group and has published systematic reviews and meta-analyses on urinary incontinence in men and women. With commitment to training and education, Ammar has the Assigned Educational Supervisory role within the East of Scotland Training Programme in Urology, he is also the Associate Editor for BJUI Knowledge on Reconstructive Urology, Female Urology and Urodynamics. He is also the module lead for reconstructive urology on the ChM in Urology course at the Royal College of Surgeons of Edinburgh and the University of Edinburgh.

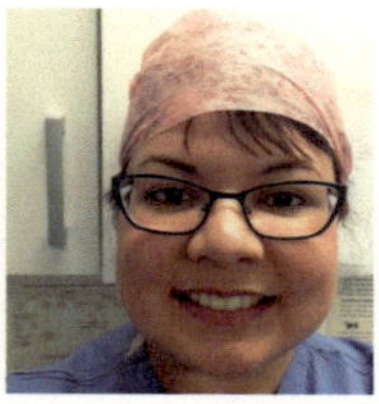

Holly Bekarma FRCS Urol graduated from the University of Manchester and is a final year Urology Registrar in the West of Scotland. She has developed a sub-specialist interest in female urology and the management of incontinence. Ms Bekarma has authored several peer reviewed publications, book chapters and presented widely on a national and international level on the topics of urinary incontinence, vaginal mesh complications and oncology. Ms Bekarma is actively involved in medical education and is presently undertaking a Master's degree from the University of Glasgow, investigating the impact of gender on self-assessment within urology trainees.

Contents

Preface

The prevalence of urinary incontinence increases with age. It has recognised social and psychological impact on individuals as well as a financial implication to individuals and healthcare systems.

The book attempt to discuss the assessment of urinary incontinence, followed by surgical and conservative treatment options in a concise way, within the framework of clinical practice.

We would like to acknowledge all the authors for their hard work in completing this book.

Ammar Alhasso
MBChB, MSc surgical Sciences, FRCSEd (UROL)
Consultant Urological Surgeon in Reconstructive Urology,
Female Urology and Urodynamics
Honorary Clinical Senior Lecturer at the University of Edinburgh, UK

Holly Bekarma
MBChB, FRCS (UROL)
Specialist Registrar in Urological Surgery,
subspecialisation in Female Urology and Urodynamics
West Scotland Training Progreamme in Urology, Glasgow, UK

Section 1

Assessment

Chapter 1

Assessment of Urinary Incontinence (UI) in Adult Patients

Raheela M. Rizvi and Mohammad Hammad Ather

Additional information is available at the end of the chapter

http://dx.doi.org/10.5772/66953

Abstract

The diagnosis and assessment of urinary incontinence (UI) are variable. In general, diagnosis is made in primary care using clinical evaluation (a good history and physical examination), bladder diary and validated symptom scales. Condition-specific diagnosis is made in secondary care, and it often involves interventional tools such as urodynamic studies. The evidence available on the accuracy and acceptability of the assessment of UI is inconsistent and variable. A structured data collection tool was used for initial assessment of UI. Some key questions are required for initial assessment of UI in order to diagnose the type of UI. This chapter includes a gender-specific evaluation based on history and clinical examination. Pelvic organ prolapse (POP) in female patients is associated with UI and POP diagnosis, and staging is made by clinical examination only, while male patients are examined for prostate obstructive urinary symptoms. Basic evaluation includes bladder diary in cases of overactive bladder and stress test, for stress urinary incontinence. Other diagnostic tests include urine analysis, uroflowmetry and measurement of post-void residual volume in cases of neurogenic bladder and benign prostate hypertrophy. Patients referred to specialist require further assessment of UI using urodynamic testing, electrophysiological test and imaging.

Keywords: assessment, adult, male, female, urinary incontinence

1. Introduction

Urinary incontinence (UI), the involuntary leakage of urine, often remains undetected and undertreated [1]. Estimates of prevalence vary depending on the population studied and the instruments used to assess severity. The prevalence of UI increases with age. Women are generally reluctant to initiate discussions about their incontinence and urinary symptoms due to embarrassment, lack of knowledge about treatment options and/or fear of surgery.

The objectives of initial assessment are to establish a presumptive or disease-specific diagnosis by excluding other conditions that mimic UI. The treatment is offered according to the level of bother and impact of UI on patient's quality of life (QoL). A detailed assessment is required to initiate initial treatment or to plan complex testing, which may require specialist referral. It also aids in the assessment of the level of improvement after any intervention from information obtained from patient or care providers.

A critical step in the evaluation of urinary incontinence is the use of up-to-date terminology to describe different types of UI and their associated lower urinary tract symptoms (LUTS). LUTS includes both storage and emptying symptoms in distinction to overactive bladder syndrome (OAB) that describes the subset of storage symptoms urgency, frequency and nocturia with or without the symptoms of UI.

The terminology defined below is adopted from a review available from the 5th International Consultation on Incontinence [2]. The use of standardized terminology during the taking of the history of the types of UI ensures uniformity in the assessment of symptoms that lead to diagnose various types of UI.

Male LUTS are a frequently encountered constellation of symptoms that consist of both storage and emptying functions of the lower tract. The index male patient with LUTS is either an elderly male with bothersome dysfunction of storage, voiding and/or the post-micturition period that often consists of a combination of frequency, urgency, nocturia, as well as hesitancy, weak stream and feeling of incomplete emptying. The other index male patient is a young male with mostly storage symptoms and sometimes voiding as well.

2. Terminology

Stress urinary incontinence (SUI) is referred to as involuntary urinary loss of effort or physical exertion, e.g. sporting activities or of sneezing or coughing.

Urgency urinary incontinence (UUI) is a condition referred to as involuntary loss of urine associated with a desire to void.

Postural urinary incontinence is a condition of involuntary loss of urine associated with change of body position, e.g. rising from a seated or lying position.

Mixed urinary incontinence (MUI) is the complaint of involuntary loss of urine associated with urgency and also with exertion, effort, sneezing or coughing.

Incontinence associated with chronic retention of urine is defined as a complaint of involuntary loss of urine, which occurs in conditions where the bladder does not empty completely as indicated by a significantly high residual urine volume and/or a non-painful bladder, which remains palpable or percussable after the individual has passed urine. (Note: The International Continence Society (ICS) no longer recommends the term overflow incontinence. A significant residual urine volume denotes a minimum volume of 300 mL, although this figure has not been well established).

Nocturnal enuresis: Complaint of involuntary loss of urine that occurs during sleep.

Continuous (urinary) incontinence: Complaint of constant involuntary loss of urine.

Insensible (urinary) incontinence: Complaint of urinary incontinence where the individual is unaware of how it occurred, the first sensation of which is a feeling of being wet.

Coital incontinence (for women only): Complaint of involuntary loss of urine with coitus. This symptom can be further divided into that occurring with penetration or intromission and that occurring at orgasm.

Functional incontinence: Complaint of involuntary loss of urine that results from an inability to reach the toilet due to cognitive, functional or mobility impairments in the presence of an intact lower urinary tract system.

Post-prostatectomy incontinence (PPI) generally is used for stress urinary incontinence following radical prostatectomy for prostate cancer. However, the term is also used for post-transurethral prostatectomy for benign prostate hypertrophy (BPH). Although small degrees of incidental incontinence may go virtually unnoticed, larger degrees of incontinence can have a major impact on a man's quality of life.

2.1. Bladder storage symptoms

Bladder storage symptoms are experienced during the bladder filling.

Increased daytime urinary frequency: Complaint that micturition occurs more frequently during waking hours than previously deemed normal. Traditionally, seven episodes of micturition during waking hours were considered as the upper limit of normal, although it may be higher in some populations.

Nocturia: Complaint of interruption of sleep one or more times because of the need to void. Each void is preceded and followed by sleep. (Note: The number of nocturia episodes and the degree of bother based on number have been questioned and the threshold of 2–3 per night has been suggested.) [3–5].

Urgency: Complaint of a sudden, compelling desire to pass urine, which is difficult to defer (Note: The 'all or none' nature of 'urgency' has been questioned.) [6].

Overactive bladder syndrome (OAB): Urinary urgency, usually accompanied by increased urinary frequency and nocturia, with or without urgency urinary incontinence, in the absence of urinary tract infection (UTI) or other obvious pathology.

2.2. Diagnostic evaluation

2.2.1. History and physical examination

The initial assessment includes a very good history and the use of validated questionnaire to know the type of urinary incontinence and its impact on patient's quality of life (QoL). A detailed history enables to diagnose complicated cases of UI-like UI associated with pelvic organ prolapse (POP), MUI, neurogenic bladder dysfunction and continuous UI secondary to diverticulum or fistula.

A good history should also identify patients who need rapid referral to an appropriate specialist. These include patients with associated pain, haematuria, history of recurrent urinary tract infection (UTI), pelvic surgery (particularly pelvic organ prolapse surgery) and UI associated with known abnormality of the urinary tract. Women with obstetric history including complicated labour followed by continuous UI are suggestive of a fistula. A detailed gynaecological history may help to understand the underlying cause, for example, polycystic ovarian disease and associated insulin resistance leading to UI among women of younger age group [7].

The medical history should include history of smoking and chronic cough, chronic obstructive pulmonary disease (COPD), congestive heart failure and diabetes. A poor glycaemic control and medication for cardiac disease are associated with UI.

Use of questionnaires may facilitate disclosure of embarrassing symptoms, ensure that symptoms are not omitted and standardize information for audit and research. In the absence of questionnaire use, **Table 1** summarizes key questions for the initial assessment of urinary incontinence.

The International Modular Questionnaire (ICIQ) was developed to meet the need of a universally acceptable standard guide for the selection of questionnaires to be used in clinical practice and research [8]. Urine output is greatly dependent upon the quantity and type of fluids taken during the day. Patients' record of volume and frequency of micturition provides an excellent record for discrimination of the physiologic influences on the pattern and frequency of micturition. This is called frequency volume charting. Use of additional information like

Do you leak urine?
If yes then do you feel the leak of urine?
If yes then does it occur with urgency and on the way to toilet? (Identify trigger factor such as key in latch.)
Do you wake up at night to void, if yes then how frequent?
If urinary leak is without sensation then questions related to neurological/cognitive deficits should be asked co-existing diseases (diabetes, heart disease, neurological impairment should be ruled out).
Do you leak urine when you cough, sneeze, laugh and during physical exertion? (Identify circumstances, e.g. sexual activity, posture change.)
Duration of the symptoms?
Frequency of leak accidents and the amount of leak.
Associated symptoms of pelvic organ prolapse (POP), fecal incontinence (FI) should be asked along with identification of risk factors as complicated deliveries, pelvic surgery, and chronic constipation.
Impact on personal and social life?
Episodes of urinary tract infection or haematuria?

Table 1. Key questions in the` initial assesment of urinary incontinence.

http://dx.doi.org/10.5772/66953

fluid intake, use of pads, activities during recording or symptom scores constitutes the bladder diary. It is recommended by European Association of Urology (EAU) guidelines that micturition frequency volume charts (FVCs) or bladder diaries should be used to assess male LUTS with a prominent storage component or nocturia. It is also recommended that these records be performed for at least 3 days for validation. Each module provides questions related to core symptoms and impact on health-related quality of life (HRQL). ICIQ provides evaluation of lower urinary tract symptoms (LUTS), urinary incontinence, vaginal symptoms and bowel symptoms although more extensive information can be found on www.iciq.net.

The International Prostate Symptom Score (IPSS) is an eight-item questionnaire, consisting of seven symptom questions and one quality-of-life question [9]. The IPSS score is used to categorize patients into four categories. This is helpful in deciding about treatment strategy. The categorization is 'asymptomatic' (0 points), 'mildly symptomatic' (1–7 points), 'moderately symptomatic' (8–19 points) and 'severely symptomatic' (20–35 points). There are many limitations to the use of IPSS, and these include lack of assessment of incontinence, of post-micturition symptoms and of bother caused by each separate symptom. Another limitation is that a basic minimum education level is required for filling the form. An alternate to this is a use of Visual prostate symptom score (VPSS), which is visual counterpart of the IPSS [10].

The International Consultation on Incontinence Questionnaire for Male LUTS (ICIQ-MLUTS) was created from the ICS male questionnaire. It is a widely used and validated patient completed questionnaire [11]. It contains 13 items, with subscales for nocturia and OAB, and is available in 17 languages [12]. The EAU guidelines recommend that a validated symptom score questionnaire including QoL assessment should be used during the assessment of male LUTS and for re-evaluation during and/or after treatment [12].

A clinical examination remains an essential part of the assessment of patients with UI. It is essential that all patient presented with UI should be mentally competent and be capable of independent toileting.

A careful abdominal examination should be performed for surgical scars, hernias, masses, organomegaly and distended bladder after voiding. The presence of hernias may indicate inherent connective tissue weakness, a possible contributor to incontinence. Masses may contribute to stress incontinence and, occasionally, may cause obstructed voiding with resultant overflow incontinence.

Pelvic examination should be performed as a routine gynaecological examination. It begins with the inspection of the external genitalia and urethral meatus. Evidence of atrophy, such as pallor and thinness of tissue, may indicate oestrogen deficiency. A red, fleshy lesion of the posterior urethra, a caruncle, may be another indicator of urogenital hypoestrogenism. The suburethral area should be inspected and palpated. A suburethral mass should raise suspicion for a urethral diverticulum. Any pelvic floor defect should be documented using pelvic organ prolapse (POP) grading. For standardization and uniformity in staging the degree of prolapse, it is recommended that pelvic organ prolapse quantification (POP-Q) method should be used as shown in **Figure 1** [13]. POP-Q involves measurement of both anterior and posterior vaginal walls and cervical prolapse with reference to hymen and defines four stages of POP as shown in **Figure 2** [13].

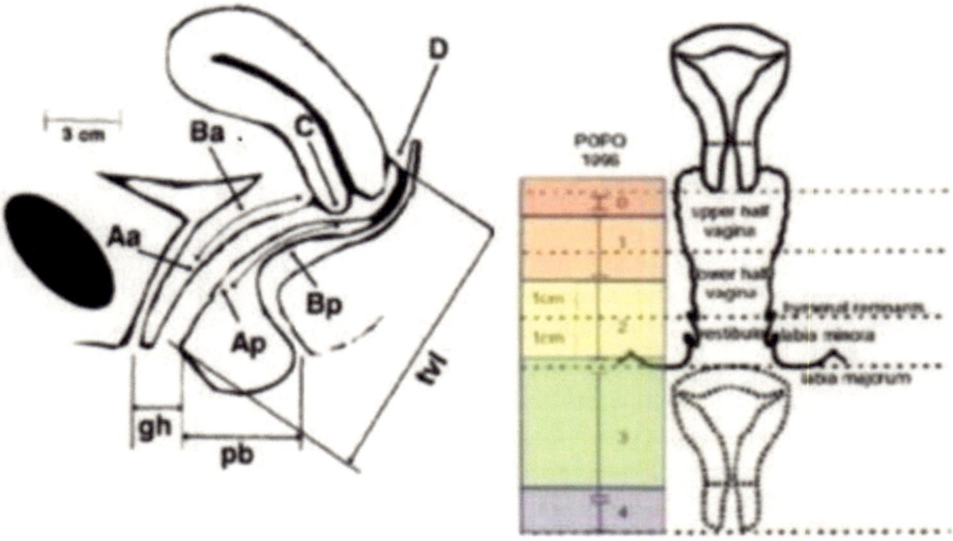

Figure 1. Pelvic organ prolapse quantification.

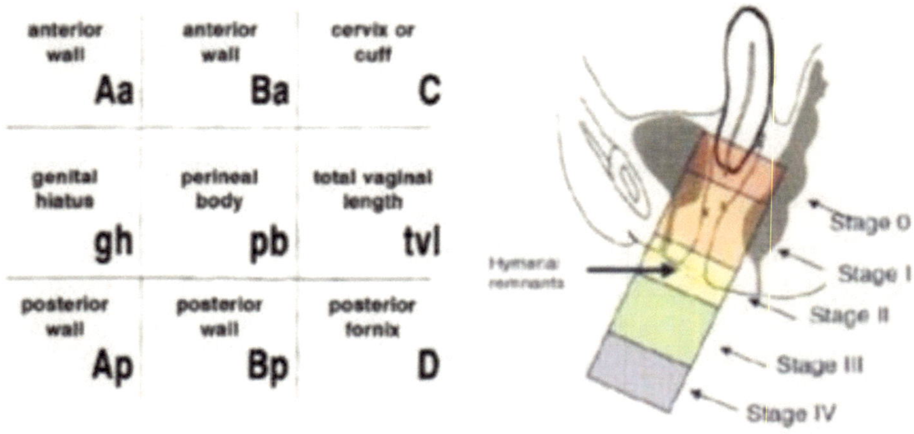

Figure 2. POP-Q staging.

2.2.2. Stress test

A cough test should be performed with comfortably full bladder in standing position and it may reveal SUI. Price and Noblett recently compared the accuracy of the cough stress to the pad test for diagnosing stress urinary incontinence [14]. The cough stress test demonstrated

http://dx.doi.org/10.5772/66953

superiority over the pad test with a sensitivity, specificity and positive and negative predictive values of 90, 80, 98 and 44%, respectively, for diagnosing stress urinary incontinence. A negative test is less useful because a false negative may result from a small urine volume in the bladder or from patient inhibition.

2.2.3. *Q-tip test*

This test is not routinely performed, and it was used to assess urethral hypermobility (also referred to as bladder neck hypermobility), present in most women who have primary SUI. Historically, the urethral cotton swab test (Q-tip test) was the most common test used to evaluate urethral mobility; it has questionable test-retest and inter-observer reliability [15]. Studies have demonstrated that almost all (over 90%) women with advanced point Aa prolapse will have a positive cotton swab test [16]. The role of urethral hypermobility testing is currently limited as it is unlikely to change management.

2.2.4. *Examination of prostate*

Men with BPH often present with paradoxical incontinence. Paradoxical incontinence or overflow incontinence is a condition, which clinically presents with UI, however, these patients are in urinary retention. The assessment of these patients often starts with physical examination following a careful history. The key to diagnosis is the presence of palpable bladder with prostomegaly.

Determination of prostate volume is important to give an idea about the presence of prostatic enlargement and its presumed aetiology for obstruction. In men with symptoms suggestive of BPH, an accurate estimation of the degree of prostate volume enlargement is important for the choice of treatment, and for prediction of the treatment effect, the risk of acute urinary retention and the need for surgery. Digital-rectal examination (DRE) is the simplest way to assess prostate volume; however, its correlation with actual volume as determined by transrectal ultrasound (TRUS) is rather poor. DRE underestimates the prostate volume particularly with volume >30 mL [17]. A model of visual aids has been developed to help urologists estimate prostate volume more accurately [18]. One study concluded that DRE was sufficient to discriminate between prostate volumes more or less than 50 mL [19].

2.2.5. *Pelvic assessment*

Pelvic floor muscle contraction should be assessed by digital posterior vaginal wall examination, and any pelvic floor muscle dysfunction should be documented using the International Continence Society (ICS) terminology [20].

2.2.6. *Neurological examination*

A detailed neurological examination is not necessary in the initial evaluation of all women with incontinence unless patients present with sudden onset of incontinence (especially urgency symptoms) or new onset of neurologic symptoms [21]. In patients where there is a concern for neurological disease, a limited evaluation of lower extremity strength, reflexes and perineal sensation is required. Unilateral weakness or hyper-reflexia of the lower extremity may identify an upper motor lesion. Absent perineal sensation with decreased rectal tone is concerning for cauda equina syndrome.

2.2.7. Pad testing

Pad test is not routinely performed, and it is part of research studies only. Measurement of urine loss using an absorbent pad worn over a set period of time or during a protocol of physical exercise can be used to quantify the presence and severity of UI, and of response to treatment. The usefulness of pad tests in quantifying severity and predicting outcome of treatment is uncertain [22]. There is no evidence that one type of pad test is superior to another.

2.2.8. Voiding diaries

Voiding diaries include information on incontinence episodes, pad usage, fluid intake, degree of urgency and degree of UI. Several studies have compared patients' preference for, and the accuracy of, electronic and paper voiding diaries in voiding dysfunction [23–26]. A recent guideline on urinary incontinence by European Association of Urology recommends that patients with urinary incontinence should be asked to complete a voiding diary for 3–7 days to evaluate co-existing storage and voiding dysfunction. It is recommended by EAU guidelines that micturition frequency volume charts or bladder diaries should be used to assess male LUTS with a prominent storage component or nocturia. It is also recommended that these records be performed for at least 3 days for validation [27]. The ideal duration of a diary is not clear; however, 5th ICI recommends 1-day frequency volume chart (FVC) which includes the first morning void the following day as a reasonable tool to gain insight into voiding habits during normal daily routine [2].

2.3. Laboratory tests

Only a few clinical tests are necessary for the initial evaluation of a woman with urinary incontinence, as conservative treatment can be initiated based on the symptoms alone.

A urinalysis should be performed in all patients, and urine culture performed if a urinary tract infection (UTI) is suggested on screening. Urinalysis (dipstick or sediment) must be included in the primary evaluation of any patient presenting with LUTS to identify conditions, such as urinary tract infections (UTI), non-visible haematuria and diabetes mellitus. Urinalysis is recommended in most guidelines in the primary management of patients with LUTS [28, 29]. There is a limited evidence, yet general expert consensus that the benefits outweigh the costs [30]. The value of urinary dipstick/microscopy for diagnosing UTI in men with LUTS without acute frequency and dysuria has recently been questioned [31].

Urine cytology is indicated in patients without UTI who have visible or non-visible haematuria with risk factors for malignancy (e.g. extensive smoking history). Renal function tests are not required unless there is a concern for severe urinary retention resulting in hydronephrosis [32]. Other laboratory testing is determined by signs or symptoms elicited in history and physical exam.

http://dx.doi.org/10.5772/66953

2.3.1. Post-void residual

Female patients who present with storage-specific symptoms, with normal sensation and no complaints of decreased bladder emptying, and no anatomical, neurological, organ-specific or co-morbid risk factors for retention may not require the measurement of PVR urine. A PVR should be performed when decreased bladder emptying is suspected in patients with neurologic disease, recurrent urinary tract infections, history concerning for detrusor under activity or bladder outlet obstruction (BOO), history of urinary retention, severe constipation, pelvic organ prolapse beyond the hymen, new onset or recurrent incontinence after surgery for incontinence, diabetes mellitus with peripheral neuropathy or medications that suppress bladder contractility or increase sphincter tone [2].

PVR is assessed by transabdominal ultrasound, bladder scan or catheterization. Jalbani and Ather [33] noted that the bladder scan estimate is as accurate as catheterization for determining the PVR urinary volume. Its accuracy was also comparable when the urinary volume is <100 mL, and there was no significant effect of age, gender and body mass index. This system could replace the more invasive catheterization with excellent accuracy. High PVR is either due to obstruction (like benign prostatic obstruction, BPO, in ageing men) or poor detrusor contraction (frequently seen in diabetics). Higher PVRs are reliable marker for BPO. Two landmark studies, i.e. medical therapy of prostate symptoms (MTOPSs) and alfuzosin long-term efficacy and safety study (ALTESS) have assessed the impact of significant PVR and risk of disease progression. Both the medical therapy of prostate symptoms (MTOPSs) and alfuzosin long-term efficacy and safety study (ALTESS) studies showed that high baseline PVR is associated with increased risk of symptom progression [34, 35].

2.3.2. Role of Urodynamic

Urodynamic studies are defined as a functional study of lower urinary tract. It is an invasive procedure and includes filling and voiding cystometry, pressure flow studies, urethral sphincter electromyography (EMG), urethral function tests/urethral pressure profilometry and videourodynamics (VUDS). These studies involve the use of a double- or triple-lumen urethral catheter to fill the bladder and record bladder and urethral pressures (need triple-lumen catheter). Detrusor pressures are not directly measured. It is a calculated value for intra-bladder pressure (determined by bladder catheter) minus the intra-abdominal pressure (determined by rectal catheter).

It is not required in the initial evaluation of urinary incontinence in women whose symptoms are consistent with stress, urgency or mixed, incontinence [36]. A 2013 systematic review of 99 studies including over 80,000 women found that urodynamic testing can establish the diagnosis of urodynamic stress urinary incontinence but it cannot predict the outcome of surgical treatment [37]. A detailed account of commonly performed urodynamic testing is given below:

2.3.2.1. Uroflowmetry

Uroflowmetry provides a non-invasive easy to perform test to assess the dynamics of urinary flow. The amount of information provided by UFM, along with ultrasonic estimation of residual urine in the bladder, usually is enough in the routine evaluation of elderly men with lower urinary tract symptoms (LUTS). It is one of the most common performed urodynamic studies. The common clinical parameters used to assess the flow dynamics include maximum flow rate (Qmax) and flow pattern [38]. The diagnostic accuracy of uroflowmetry for detecting BPO is variable and is substantially influenced by threshold values. A threshold Qmax of 10 mL/s has a specificity of 70%, a PPV of 70% and a sensitivity of 47% for BOO. The specificity using a threshold Qmax of 15 mL/s was 38%, the PPV 67% and the sensitivity 82% [39].The main limitation of UFM is its inability to discriminate between poor detrusor function and bladder outlet obstruction (BOO), for which pressure flow studies are necessary.

2.3.2.2. Filling and voiding cystometry

Table 2 summarizes the indications for urodynamic studies comprising of filling and voiding cystometry.

Severe stress incontinence, previous pelvic radiation, previous anti-incontinence surgery
Overactive bladder not responding to conservative therapy
UI with voiding dysfunction
Voiding difficulty associated with UI and POP
Poorly definable or inconclusive history to support UI
Associated with diseases, which can affect the function of LUT/pelvic floor, e.g. diabetes mellitus, Parkinson's disease, cerebrovascular accident and prolapsed intervertebral disc

Table 2. Indications for urodynamic studies.

2.3.2.3. Ambulatory and videourodynamics

Ambulatory and videourodynamics are indicated only if the diagnosis is unclear after conventional urodynamics [40].

2.3.3. MRI Pelvic floor ultrasound and EMG

Imaging improves our understanding of the anatomical and functional abnormalities that may cause UI. In clinical research, MRI and EMG are used to evaluate urethral support in cases of SUI. There is a general consensus that MRI provides good global pelvic floor assessment, including POP, defecatory function and integrity of the pelvic floor support [32]. However, it is not considered useful in the evaluation of UI [33]. Ultrasound imaging can reliably be used to measure bladder neck and urethral mobility in cases of SUI but it is not routinely performed in the initial assessment of UI.

3. Conclusions

Urinary incontinence is of various types, and its initial assessment requires detailed history taking and clinical examination. Since the disease has major impact on patient's quality of

http://dx.doi.org/10.5772/66953

life hence the evaluation should lead to establish types of UI. Very few patients need invasive testing and usually urine analysis, culture, bladder diary, stress test are enough for initial assessment. Patients with neurogenic bladder and overactive bladder syndrome need specific testing for final diagnosis.

Author details

Raheela M. Rizvi[1]* and Mohammad Hammad Ather[2]

*Address all correspondence to: raheela.mohsin@aku.edu

1 Department of Obstetrics and Gynecology, Aga Khan University, Karachi, Pakistan

2 Department of Surgery, Aga Khan University, Karachi, Pakistan

References

[1] Abrams P, Cardozo L, Fall M, Griffiths D, Rosier P, Ulmsten U, van Kerrebroeck P, Victor A, Wein A. The standardisation of terminology of lower urinary tract function: report from the Standardisation Sub-committee of the International Continence Society. Standardisation Sub-committee of the International Continence Society. Neurourol Urodyn. 2002;21(2):167–78.

[2] Andersson KE, Chapple CR, Cardozo L, Cruz F, Hashim H, Michel MC, Abrams P, Khoury S, Wein AJ. Incontinence, 5th International Consultation on Incontinence. Abrams P, Cardozo L, Khoury S, Wein AJ [Paris]: ICUD-EAU. 2013:623–728.

[3] Tikkinen KAO, Johnson TM, Tammela RLJ, et al. Nocturia frequency, bother and quality of life: how often is too often? A population-based study in Finland. Eur Urol. 2010;57:488–98.

[4] Kim SO, Choi HS, Kim YJ, Kim HS, Hwang IS, Hwang EC, Oh KJ, Jung SI, Kang TW, Kwon D, Park K, Ryu SB. Impact of nocturia on health-related quality of life and medical outcomes study sleep score in men. Int Neurourol J. 2011;15(2):82–6.

[5] Vaughan CP, Eisenstein R, Bliwise DL, Endeshaw YK, Nagamia ZJ, Wolf RA, Johnson TM. Self-rated sleep characteristics and bother from nocturia. Int J Clin Pract. 2012;66(4):369–73.

[6] De Wachter S, Hanno P. Urgency: all or none phenomenon? Neurourol Urodyn. 2010; 29:616–7.

[7] Uzun H, Yilmaz A, Kemik A, Zorba OU, Kalkan M. Association of insulin resistance with overactive bladder in female patients. Int Neurourol J. 2012;16(4):181–6.

[8] Avery K, Donovan J, Peters TJ, et al. ICIQ: a brief and robust measure for evaluating the symptoms and impact of urinary incontinence. Neurourol Urodyn. 2004;23(4):322–30.

[9] Barry, MJ, et al. The American Urological Association symptom index for benign prostatic hyperplasia. The Measurement Committee of the American Urological Association. J Urol. 1992;148:1549.

[10] Memon MA, Ather MH. Relationship between visual prostate score (VPSS) and maximum flow rate (Qmax) in men with urinary tract symptoms. Int Braz J Urol. 2016;42(2):321–6.

[11] Donovan, JL, et al. Scoring the short form ICS male SF questionnaire. International Continence Society. J Urol. 2000;164:1948.

[12] Gravas S, Bach T, Bachmann A, Drake M, Gacci M, Gratzke C. EAU guidelines on the management of non-neurogenic male lower urinary tract symptoms (LUTS), incl. benign prostatic obstruction (BPO) 2016.

[13] Lemos N, Korte JE, Iskander M, Freeman R, Arunkalaivanan A, Rizk D, Halaska M, Medina C, Conceição JC, Parekh M, Martan A. Center-by-center results of a multicenter prospective trial to determine the inter-observer correlation of the simplified POP-Q in describing pelvic organ prolapse. International urogynecology journal. 2012 May 1;23(5):579–84.

[14] Price DM, Noblett K. Comparison of the cough stress test and 24-h pad test in the assessment of stress urinary incontinence. International urogynecology journal. 2012 Apr 1;23(4):429–33.

[15] Swift S, Barnes D, Herron A, Goodnight W. Test-retest reliability of the cotton swab (Q-tip) test in the evaluation of the incontinent female. Int Urogynecol J. 2010;21(8):963.

[16] Mattison ME, Simsiman AJ, Menefee SA. Can urethral mobility be assessed using the pelvic organ prolapse quantification system? An analysis of the correlation between point Aa and Q-tip angle in varying stages of prolapse. Urology. 2006;68(5):1005.

[17] Roehrborn CG. Accurate determination of prostate size via digital rectal examination and transrectal ultrasound. Urology. 1998;51(4A Suppl):19–22.

[18] Roehrborn CG, Sech S, Montoya J, Rhodes T, Girman CJ. Interexaminer reliability and validity of a three-dimensional model to assess prostate volume by digital rectal examination. Urology. 2001;57(6):1087–92.

[19] Bosch JL, Bohnen AM, Groeneveld FP. Validity of digital rectal examination and serum prostate specific antigen in the estimation of prostate volume in community-based men aged 50 to 78 years: the Krimpen Study. Eur Urol. 2004;46(6):753–9.

[20] Messelink B, Benson T, Berghmans B, et al. Standardization of terminology of pelvic floor muscle function and dysfunction: report from the Pelvic Floor Clinical Assessment Group of the International Continence Society. Neurourol Urodyn. 2005;24:374–80.

[21] Staskin D, Hilton P, Emmanuel A, et al. Initial assessment of incontinence. In: Incontinence: 3rd International Consultation on Incontinence, Abrams P, Cardozo L, Khoury S, Wein A (Eds), Health Publications Ltd, Paris, France 2005. p. 485.

[22] Al Afraa TA, et al. Normal lower urinary tract assessment in women: uroflowmetry and post-void residual, pad tests, and bladder diaries. Int Urogynecol J. 2012;23(6):681–5.

[23] Quinn P, et al. Assessment of an electronic daily diary in patients with overactive bladder. BJU Int. 2003;91(7):647–52.

[24] Rabin JM, et al. Computerized voiding diary. Neurourol Urodyn. 1993;12(6):541–53; discussion 553–4.

[25] Rabin JM, et al. A computerized voiding diary. J Reprod Med. 1996;41(11):801–6.

[26] Rabin JM, et al. "Compu-Void II": the computerized voiding diary. J Med Syst. 1996;20(1):19–34.

[27] Lucas MG, Bedretdinova D, Berghmans LC, Bosch HR, Burkhard FC, Cruz F, Nambiar AK, Nilsson CG, Tubaro A, Pickard RS. Guidelines on Urinary Incontinence. European Association of Urology.UK 2015.

[28] Roehrborn CG, Bartsch G, Kirby R, Andriole G, Boyle P, de la Rosette J, Perrin P, Ramsey E, Nordling J, De Campos Freire G, Arap S. Guidelines for the diagnosis and treatment of benign prostatic hyperplasia: a comparative, international overview. Urology. 2001;58(5):642–50.

[29] Abrams P, Chapple C, Khoury S, Roehrborn C, de la Rosette J. International Consultation on New Developments in Prostate Cancer and Prostate Diseases. Evaluation and treatment of lower urinary tract symptoms in older men. J Urol. 2013;189(1 Suppl):S93–101. doi: 10.1016/j.juro.2012.11.021.

[30] European Confederation of Laboratory Medicine. European urinalysis guidelines. Scand J Clin Lab Invest Suppl. 2000;231:1–86.

[31] Khasriya R, Khan S, Lunawat R, Bishara S, Bignall J, Malone-Lee M, Ishii H, O'Connor D, Kelsey M, Malone-Lee J. The inadequacy of urinary dipstick and microscopy as surrogate markers of urinary tract infection in urological outpatients with lower urinary tract symptoms without acute frequency and dysuria. J Urol. 2010;183(5):1843–7. doi: 10.1016/j.juro.2010.01.008. Epub 2010 Mar 29.

[32] Abrams P, Andersson KE, Birder L, Brubaker L, Cardozo L, Chapple C, Cottenden A, Davila W, de Ridder D, Dmochowski R, Drake M, Dubeau C, Fry C, Hanno P, Smith JH, Herschorn S, Hosker G, Kelleher C, Koelbl H, Khoury S, Madoff R, Milsom I, Moore K, Newman D, Nitti V, Norton C, Nygaard I, Payne C, Smith A, Staskin D, Tekgul S, Thuroff J, Tubaro A, Vodusek D, Wein A, Wyndaele JJ, Members of Committees. Fourth International Consultation on Incontinence. Neurourol Urodyn. 2010;29(1):213–40.

[33] Jalbani IK, Ather MH. The accuracy of three-dimensional bladder ultrasonography in determining the residual urinary volume compared with conventional catheterisation. Arab J Urol. 2014;12(3):209–13.

[34] McConnell JD1, Roehrborn CG, Bautista OM, Andriole GL Jr, Dixon CM, Kusek JW, Lepor H, McVary KT, Nyberg LM Jr, Clarke HS, Crawford ED, Diokno A, Foley JP, Foster HE, Jacobs SC, Kaplan SA, Kreder KJ, Lieber MM, Lucia MS, Miller GJ, Menon M, Milam DF, Ramsdell JW, Schenkman NS, Slawin KM, Smith JA; Medical Therapy of Prostatic Symptoms (MTOPS) Research Group. The long-term effect of doxazosin, finasteride, and combination therapy on the clinical progression of benign prostatic hyperplasia. N Engl J Med. 2003;349(25):2387–98.

[35] Roehrborn CG. Alfuzosin 10 mg once daily prevents overall clinical progression of benign prostatic hyperplasia but not acute urinary retention: results of a 2-year placebo-controlled study. BJU Int. 2006;97(4):734–41.

[36] Winters JC, Dmochowski RR, Goldman HB, Herndon CD, Kobashi KC, Kraus SR, Lemack GE, Nitti VW, Rovner ES, Wein AJ, Urodynamic studies in adults: AUA/SUFU guideline. American Urological Association, Society of Urodynamics, Female Pelvic Medicine & Urogenital Reconstruction. J Urol. 2012;188(6 Suppl):2464–72.

[37] Hang AJ. Nonsurgical treatments for urinary incontinence in women: summary of primary findings and conclusions. JAMA Intern Med. 2013;173(15):1463.

[38] Ather MH, Memon A. Uroflowmetry and evaluation of voiding disorders. Tech Urol. 1998;4(3):111–7.

[39] Reynard JM, Yang Q, Donovan JL, Peters TJ, Schafer W, de la Rosette JJ, Dabhoiwala NF, Osawa D, Lim AT, Abrams P. The ICS-'BPH' Study: uroflowmetry, lower urinary tract symptoms and bladder outlet obstruction. Br J Urol. 1998;82(5):619–23.

[40] Nambiar AK, Lemack GE, Chapple CR, Burkhard FC, European Association of Urology. The Role of Urodynamics in the Evaluation of Urinary Incontinence: The European Association of Urology Recommendations in 2016. European Urology. 2016 Oct 7.

Section 2

Surgical Treatment

Chapter 2

Adjustable Midurethral Slings in the Treatment of Female Stress Urinary Incontinence

Funda Gungor Ugurlucan and Cenk Yasa

Additional information is available at the end of the chapter

http://dx.doi.org/10.1163/174552512X632115

Abstract

Midurethral slings have become the gold standard in the surgical treatment of stress urinary incontinence (SUI). However, despite the high cure rates with these procedures, nearly 20% of the patients are incontinent after surgery. On the other hand, in a small percentage of women, voiding dysfunction may develop after surgery. Adjustable slings have been advocated in patients who fail an anti-incontinence surgery or have intrinsic sphincter deficiency (ISD) or in order to prevent postoperative voiding dysfunction. There are various options of adjustable slings according to the surgical route or the type of mesh used.

Keywords: stress urinary incontinence, adjustable slings, midurethral slings, minisling, mesh

1. Introduction

Stress urinary incontinence (SUI) is the involuntary loss of urine occurring with increases in intra-abdominal pressure such as coughing and sneezing and is encountered in 4–35% of women [1, 2]. First-line treatments for symptomatic SUI are behavioral treatment, pelvic floor muscle exercises and continence pessaries [3]. For women who do not benefit from or are not willing to undergo conservative treatment, surgery is recommended.

In the last 20 years, there has been an increasing search and demand for minimally invasive approaches in SUI surgery. After the wide acceptance of the integral theory proposed by Petros and Ulmsten [4] suggesting that the urethral closure occurred in the midurethra, instead of suburethral slings supporting the bladder neck, midurethral slings have been developed. In 1996, Ulmsten described the tension-free vaginal tape (TVT) operation [5]. Afterward, in order to prevent potential complications of TVT, Delorme described the transobturator tape (TOT) operation in 2001 [6]. Due to their long-term efficacy, the most commonly used anti-incontinence surgeries are midurethral sling surgeries (MUS). They are similar in efficacy to conventional suburethral slings, Burch retropubic colposuspension and laparoscopic colposuspension; are minimally invasive; have shorter operating time and have less postoperative complications [3].

Midurethral slings have been classified into three generations [7]. First-generation MUS is retropubic TVT and is accepted as the gold standard surgery for SUI. Second-generation MUS is the TOT, both outside in and inside out approaches. The advantage of this technique is the avoidance of the retropubic space. Third-generation MUS are the single-incision slings, which have a shorter mesh and only a single incision that is vaginal. The long-term success rates of MUS vary between 77 and 90% [8]. Both objective and subjective success rates for single-incision slings are lower when compared to standard MUS [9].

Despite high success rates of standard MUS operations, nearly 20% of patients undergoing MUS suffer from persistent or recurrent symptoms after surgery [10, 11].Therefore, there is a need for other options in patients who fail standard minisling, transobturator, or retropubic sling operations. In addition, voiding dysfunction may develop in 2.8–38% after retropubic sling and 0–15.6% after TOT operation and additional interventions such as intermittent catheterization, sling excision and urethrolysis may be required [11].

Adjustable slings are reasonable alternatives in order to avoid or treat these two potential complications [12]. The aims of adjustable sling operations are adjusting the tension of the sling according to the severity of the patients' condition or symptoms, either during surgery or after surgery in order to prevent persistence of symptoms or development of postoperative voiding dysfunction. In some cases, there is the possibility of adjusting sling tension anytime during follow-up, even years after the primary operation. Various adjustable sling materials are discussed below according to the route of application and their adjustment techniques.

2. Adjustable slings with retropubic approach

2.1. Remeex system

Regulation Mechanical External® (Remeex; Neomedic International, Terrassa, Spain) is a readjustable sling and allows the regulation of sling tension not only in the postoperative period but also at anytime during follow-up. Theoretically, it is based on the TVT operation. The Remeex system contains 30 × 15 mm^2 type-1 macroporous polypropylene mesh, 2 polypropylene sutures attached to this mesh, a *varitensor* and a manipulator attached to the *varitensor* for the adjustment of the tension of the mesh (**Figure 1**). The *varitensor* and the manipulator are made of biocompatible materials such as titanium and ultrahigh-molecular-weight polyethylene (Chirulen®).

First, a 4 cm transverse skin incision is made 2 cm above the symphysis pubis dissecting the subcutaneous fat and exposing the rectus fascia. A vertical vaginal incision is made at

http://dx.doi.org/10.1163/174552512X632115

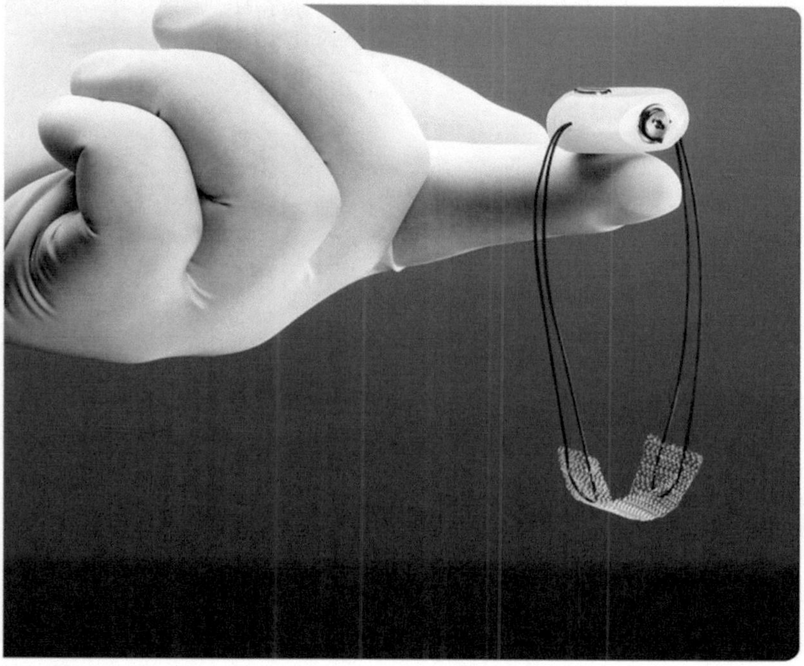

Figure 1. The Remeex system.

the level of the midurethra and dissection is continued until the pubic rami are reached. Traction needles are passed from the vaginal incision retropubically through the rectus fascia. After ensuring that the bladder is intact with cystoscopy, sutures are passed through the *varitensor* and tied (**Figure 2**). Mesh is placed at the level of the midurethra. The *varitensor* is placed over the rectus fascia and the skin and vaginal incisions are sutured. The day after surgery, the bladder is filled with 300 ml saline through the Foley catheter. The Foley catheter is removed and the patient is asked to stand up and cough. If there is any leakage, the manipulator attached to the *varitensor* can be rotated and the tension on the mesh can be adjusted. Afterward, the patient is asked to void; if the postvoid residual urine volume is less than 100 ml, the manipulator is withdrawn. If the residual urine volume is over 100 ml, the tension is decreased by rotating the manipulator on the opposite direction. If the patient develops recurrent urinary incontinence or voiding dysfunction anytime during follow-up, it is possible to incise the previous suprapubic incision under local anesthesia, find the *varitensor,* which is located inside the subcutaneous tissue and adjust the tension of the mesh by using the same technique.

Iglesias and Espuna first reported the usage of Remeex® system in 21 patients with recurrent urinary incontinence in 2003. They reported 90.5% success rate with mean follow-up of 12 months [13]. Mantovani et al. applied Remeex system in 32 patients with fixed urethra, urethral hypermobility, intrinsic sphincter deficiency (ISD) and previous anti-incontinence surgery with a follow-up of 3 years [14]. Thirty-one of the patients were cured and readjustment

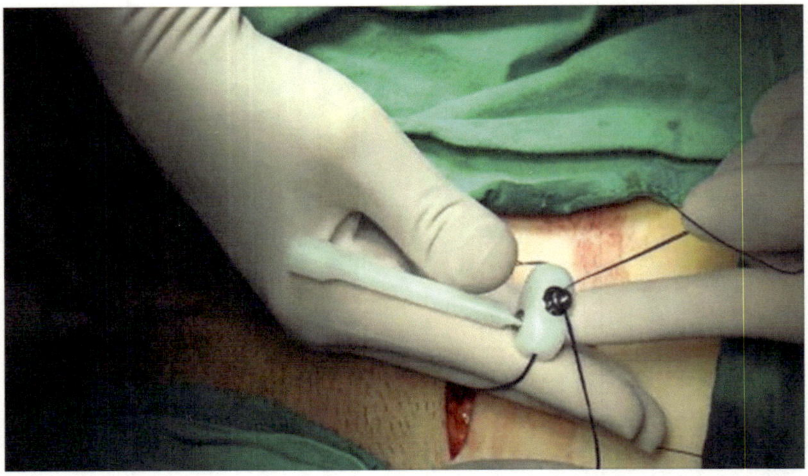

Figure 2. The Remeex system. Polypropylene sutures are passed through the *varitensor* and tied above the rectus fascia. The manipulator is attached to the *varitensor*.

was performed in three. The device was removed due to infection in one case. Yoo et al. evaluated the outcome of Remeex procedure in 17 patients in whom the success rate of tension-free slings was low, such as patients with ISD [15]. Five (29.4%) had previous anti-incontinence surgery and four (23.5%) had mixed urinary incontinence. Mean follow-up period was 13 months. Fourteen patients (82.3%) were cured and three patients (17.6%) were improved. Araco et al. applied Remeex system in 38 patients with ISD [16]. Immediate postoperative adjustment of sling tension was necessary in three patients (7.9%), two for obstructive voiding and one for incontinence. Late adjustment was necessary in three patients (7.9%), two for obstructive voiding and one for incontinence. The possibility of immediate and late adjustment of sling tension resolved postoperative failures and maintained the success rate of the Remeex system in the long term.

Moreno Sierra et al. retrospectively evaluated the outcome of Remeex system in 683 patients with mixed urinary incontinence, ISD and recurrent SUI [17]. Mean follow-up period was 23 months. 73.1% of the patients had ISD and 35.7% of the patients had a previous history of failed surgery for SUI. In this group, 92.2% cure, 6.9% improvement and 0.9% failure were observed. Errando et al., in their prospective study, evaluated the outcomes, complications and quality of life of 125 patients with recurrent SUI and ISD who underwent Remeex system [18]. After a mean follow-up of 38 months, objective and subjective cure was observed in 109 patients (87%). Sixteen patients (13%) remained incontinent, but nine (7%) were satisfied to the point that they declined readjustment of the sling. The *varitensor* was removed in one case because of infection.

Park et al. evaluated the efficacy of Remeex system in 102 patients with recurrent SUI after failed anti-incontinence surgery or ISD [19]. After a mean follow-up of 27 months, 91 patients (89.2%) were cured and six patients (5.9%) were improved. Forty percent of the patients had complications: 15 (14.7%) presented with de novo urgency, which was managed with

http://dx.doi.org/10.1163/174552512X632115

anticholinergics; 14 (13.7%) underwent delayed sling readjustment during follow-up; and six (5.9%) developed wound infection with two of these undergoing removal of the Remeex system. Although the complication rate was 40% in this study, 70% of these complications were minor and 88% of grade 3 complications were postoperative sling tension readjustments.

Yasa et al. evaluated the efficacy and safety of Remeex system in the treatment of recurrent SUI after MUS failure prospectively in 19 women [20]. Mean follow-up was 20 ± 14 months. The overall cure and improvement rates were 84.2 and 10.5%, respectively. Fifteen (79%) patients were very satisfied and three (15.7%) were moderately satisfied. Sling tension readjustment was needed during follow-up in one patient (5.3%), 13 months after the initial surgery. The authors suggested that Remeex system was effective in the treatment of recurrent SUI after MUS failure with acceptable rate of adverse effects.

Studies with long-term follow-up after Remeex procedure have been published as well. Barrington et al. evaluated the effect of Remeex system in 20 women with previous anti-incontinence surgery with a follow-up of 5 years [21]. Two systems had to be removed due to chronic infection around the *varitensor* that failed to respond to antibiotics and aspiration/drainage. However, the sling was left in situ and continence was maintained. No suture breakage or urethral erosions were observed in any patients. Two women performed intermittent self-catheterization. All the domains of the King's Health Questionnaire were improved significantly except for the general health domain at both 1 year and 5 years. There was also a significant reduction in the number of pads used daily. At 1 year, nine women considered that their incontinence had been cured by the Remeex procedure; 11 women felt their symptoms had improved. By 5 years, nine women were still cured and only two women felt the system had failed but declined any further tightening.

Giberti et al. evaluated the objective and subjective outcomes of the Remeex system for SUI caused by ISD in 30 patients, retrospectively [22]. Mean follow-up was 60.6 months. 86.0% of the patients were cured, 7.0% were improved and 7.0% had failed. There was a significant decrease in the mean pad weight and significant improvement in quality of life. Sling tension readjustment was needed in two patients (7%). Persistent urinary retention developed in 10%, seroma formation occurred in 3% and de novo urgency developed in 7% and they were treated with anticholinergics.

Main complications encountered with the Remeex system include wound infection and seroma formation, voiding dysfunction including urinary retention and de novo urge incontinence. Lorenzo-Gómez et al. evaluated the severe complications and failures of Remeex system retrospectively in 60 women [23]. The procedure was successful in 68.3% of the cases. Thirty-five percent of the patients required sling adjustment. There were three cases with severe complications: refractory urinary incontinence in one patient, massive pelvic hemorrhage in a patient who was on anticoagulant treatment and infected vaginal calculi measuring 7 cm on an eroded Remeex suture 4 years after the implantation.

All of the studies support that the Remeex system is a useful adjuvant in the treatment of recurrent or persistent SUI that has not been cured by conventional surgery. The cure rates may decline slightly over time, but this deterioration is mild and readjustment can be easily performed rather than repeating the entire sling procedure or another invasive procedure. Although this system can be used in primary surgery due to the advantage of long-term adjustability, in our opinion, it should not be used as a primary option except in cases with low urethral closing pressure, where the reported cure rates of other methods are generally lower. In addition, the procedure is more expensive than a standard TVT, but when compared to repeat surgery, it becomes cost-effective. In our opinion, it is best to perform this operation in patients with previous failed anti-incontinence procedure or ISD.

2.2. Transvaginal adjustable tape (TVA)

Transvaginal adjustable tape (TVA) (Agency for Medical Innovations, Im Letten 1, 6800 Feldkirch, Austria) insertion technique is similar to that of the TVT and suprapubic arc (SPARC) sling procedures. The tape used is a macroporous, monofilament polypropylene non-elastic mesh. Two groups of polypropylene sutures are attached to this mesh (**Figure 3**). The first group of sutures consists of two strings of polypropylene on either side situated 1.5 cm from the midline of the tape which are externalized through the vaginal wall. These sutures serve to reduce the tension on the mesh when pulled downward. The second group of sutures is formed of three strings of polypropylene in each arm of the tape situated at different distances from the midline. These are externalized from the suprapubic incisions through which the mesh is taken out. These sutures serve to increase the tension on the mesh when pulled up.

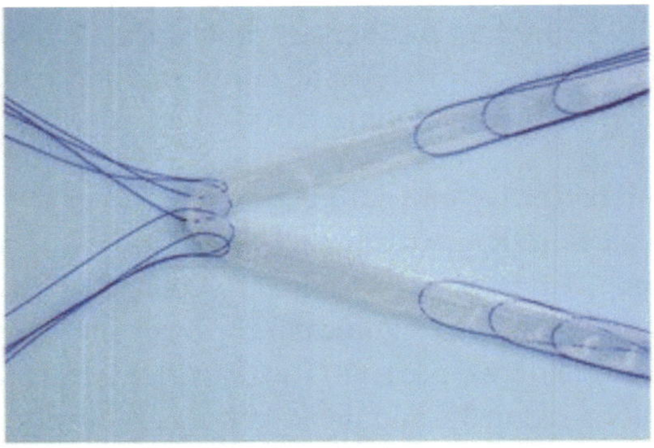

Figure 3. TVA sling [24].

Adjustment is performed the day after surgery by filling the bladder with 250 ml saline through the Foley catheter. The patient is asked to cough while standing or in the supine position. After adjustment of the tape, uroflowmetry is performed. If the maximum flow rate is below 10 ml/s or the postvoid residual urine volume is above 50 ml, the sutures on the vaginal side are pulled down in order to reduce the tension.

Romero Maroto et al. evaluated 64 women who suffered from SUI and underwent TVA prospectively [24]. Mean follow-up was 40 ± 13 months. Objective and subjective cure rates were 94 and 56%, respectively. The tension was adjusted in 26 (40.6%) patients postoperatively; in 16 (25%), the tension was increased and in 10 (15.6%), the tension was decreased. After

http://dx.doi.org/10.1163/174552512X632115

adjustment, all patients were continent and none had postvoid residual urine. Urgency disappeared or was ameliorated in 77% of cases suffering from overactive bladder symptoms preoperatively and appeared de novo in four of the 27 cases (15%). No infection and vaginal or urethral erosions were reported. There was significant improvement in quality of life. TVA mesh was found as a good option for the postoperative adjustment of tension of the mesh in patients who are incontinent after the procedure and better objective and subjective results could be obtained than those achieved with the traditional nonadjustable mesh without increasing complications. However, there are no other studies comparing TVA with other adjustable or nonadjustable slings or tapes as far as we know.

3. Adjustable slings with retropubic and transobturator approach

3.1. Safyre

Safyre (Promedon, Córdoba, Argentina) is also a type of adjustable sling used for treatment of SUI. Safyre consists of a central monofilament polypropylene mesh held between two self-anchoring columns, which are made up of polydimethylsiloxane polymer (silicone) (**Figure 4**). These columns are the basis of the adjustment system; these columns attach to the surrounding tissue and are held by fibrotic encapsulation [25]. Safyre can be inserted via retropubic approach similar to TVT or transobturator approach similar to TOT. Safyre VS, Safyre T and Safyre T Plus types can be inserted via vaginal-suprapubic, suprapubic-vaginal and transobturator routes, respectively. Intraoperative and postoperative adjustments are possible with Safyre system, but adjustments should be done under local or general anesthesia and an incision should be made in order to locate the silicone columns. The columns can be easily palpated under local anesthesia. Unilateral adjustment is usually sufficient. During this maneuver, scissors or a clamp should be inserted between the urethra and the mesh in order to avoid excessive tensioning. During adjustment, cough stress test may be used. In order to reduce the tension on the mesh, one of the arms should be held with a clamp and pulled downward. Generally, it is advised to make the adjustment within 30 days after surgery, before fibrosis occurs. However, theoretically fibrotic encapsulation of the polydimethylsiloxane columns allows easy adjustment even after this period.

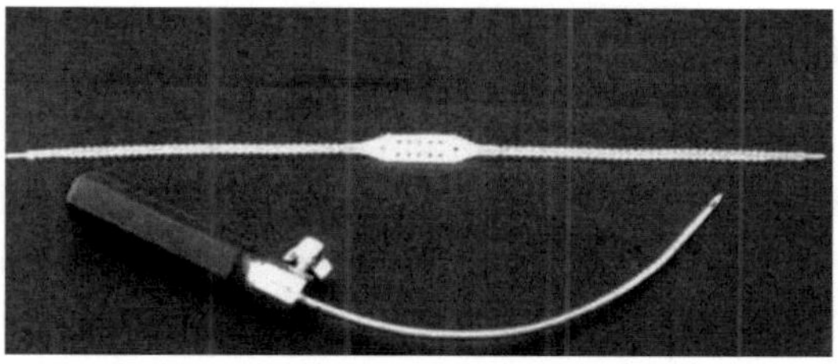

Figure 4. Safyre sling set [26].

Palma et al. reported good results with Safyre both with suprapubic and transvaginal approaches [26]. Forty-five women underwent Safyre sling operation with transvaginal approach in their preliminary prospective study [26]. Mean follow-up period was 10 months. Ninety percent of the women were continent, 3% improved and 7% were the same. Postoperative urinary retention developed in three women (6.7%) who could not void spontaneously within 4 weeks after surgery and needed sling readjustment. There were four cases (9%) of vaginal wall infection, but no vaginal or urethral wall erosion. Palma et al., in their prospective, multicenter, single-arm, unrandomized study evaluated 126 women with clinical and urodynamic SUI who underwent Safyre sling [27]. Sixty percent of the patients had a history of failed sling procedure. Mean follow-up period was 18 months. Bladder perforation developed in 2% and de novo urgency symptoms developed in 21% of the patients. Urinary retention developed in four of the 126 patients (3%) who could not void spontaneously 4 weeks after surgery and underwent sling tension loosening. During follow-up, 116 women (92%) were continent, three (2%) improved and seven (6%) were dissatisfied. Six patients (5%) presented with recurrent urinary incontinence and underwent sling adjustment. Four patients were continent afterward and symptoms improved in two. Six patients (5%) presented with vaginal pain, discharge, bleeding, dyspareunia and dysuria and were diagnosed with vaginal erosion and one had recurrent urinary tract infection. Topical treatment and oral antibiotics failed and all patients underwent transvaginal tissue debridement. The protruding part of the tape was removed in four women and reconstruction with a vaginal flap was needed in two. None of the erosions recurred. Using transobturator approach, the results were similar with a cure rate of 90% with 6 months of follow-up [28]. The same group conducted a comparative study of transobturator (n = 100) and retropubic (n = 126) approaches using Safyre in 2005 in a total of 226 patients [29]. The mean follow-up period was 18 months in the retropubic and 14 months in the transobturator group. The mean operative time was significantly longer and bladder injury was significantly greater in the retropubic group (2.3% vs 0%). There was no significant difference in the cure rate between the two groups (retropubic 92.1% and transobturator 94%). The overall complication rate was 33.3 and 20% in the retropubic and transobturator group, respectively. Postoperatively, 20.6% of the patients presented with de novo urgency in the retropubic group as opposed to 10% in the transobturator group. The authors concluded that Safyre performed by transobturator approach was as effective as the retropubic approach with the additional advantages of fewer complications and shorter operative time.

Silva-Filho et al. compared autologous pubovaginal sling with transobturator Safyre; 20 women suffering from SUI were randomly assigned to pubovaginal sling or Safyre [30]. Mean operative time and duration of hospitalization were significantly longer in the pubovaginal sling group. There were no intraoperative complications in either group. One (10%) patient in the Safyre group developed urinary retention. The mean postoperative pad test was significantly higher in the Safyre group and improvement in the quality of life parameters was better in the pubovaginal sling group. The rate of persistent SUI was significantly higher in the Safyre group (70% vs 10%). The authors ended their study prematurely due to significant discrepancy in the success rates between the two groups.

The main concerns over Safyre are the potential higher risk of erosion and dislocations due to the silicone columns. In various studies regarding urogynecologic surgery, the use of silicone

http://dx.doi.org/10.1163/174552512X632115

has been found to carry a higher risk of erosions ranging from 19 to 71% [25, 31–33]. Kuschel et al. evaluated the efficacy and safety of Safyre-t in 79 women, retrospectively [25]. The mean follow-up period was 20 ± 4 months. 59.5% of the women stated that they were subjectively continent. Vaginal sling erosion and a pre-erosive state were found in 8.8 and 13.9% of the patients, respectively. The lateral silicone column could be palpated in 47% of the patients indicating dislocation. Six women complained of dyspareunia and one woman stated that her partner had felt discomfort during sexual intercourse since her vaginal sling surgery. The authors concluded that despite acceptable subjective continence rates, Safyre-t was associated with a comparatively high rate of vaginal sling erosions and dislocations. The fibrous encapsulation of the silicone columns offers the potential advantage of adjustability but also increases the risk of dislocation. Dislocation may be related to sinus formation around the columns [32]. Padilla-Fernández et al., in their study comparing the efficacy of different types of TOT, stated that in 4 of the 44 patients who underwent Safyre implantation, the silicone column was detached from the mesh and patients had recurrent incontinence and required readjustment [34]. However, this study is limited with low numbers of patients in each mesh group.

In conclusion, Safyre, despite its advantage of intraoperative and postoperative adjustment and high subjective satisfaction rates, has shown high erosion, infection and dyspareunia rate in some studies. Comparative studies with higher number of patients and long-term follow-up are needed.

4. Adjustable slings with transobturator approach

4.1. Transobturator adjustable tape (TOA)

Transobturator adjustable tape (TOA) (Agency for Medical Innovations, Im Letten 1, 6800 Feldkirch, Austria) is a nonelastic tape made of macroporous polypropylene mesh. It contains two groups of polypropylene sutures; one group has two sutures located at 1.5 cm from the midline of the mesh laterally and is exteriorized through the anterior vaginal mucosa and used to reduce sling tension. The other group consists of three sutures in each arm of the mesh and these sutures are exteriorized through the groin incisions in order to increase the tension. Technically, the procedure is the same as the outside-in TOT.

Adjustment is performed the day after surgery by filling the bladder with 250 ml saline through the Foley catheter. The patient is asked to cough while standing or in the supine position. After adjustment of the tape by pulling the groin sutures by 0.5 cm, uroflowmetry is performed. If the maximum flow rate is below 10 ml/s or the postvoid residual urine volume is above 50 ml, the sutures on the vaginal side are pulled down in order to reduce the tension. When the adjustment is completed, the sutures are cut.

Lee et al., in their prospective multicenter study, evaluated the efficacy and safety of TOA in 65 women with SUI or combined SUI and voiding dysfunction [35]. Forty-six of the patients suffered from severe SUI and 30 patients had both SUI and voiding dysfunction. Twenty-seven of the 65 patients (41%) required tape readjustment. Fourteen patients (21%) underwent loosening and 13 patients (20%) underwent sling tensioning. Six months after surgery, the cure rate for patients with combined SUI and voiding dysfunction was 76.7% and the cure rate for patients with severe SUI was 89.1%. There was a significant improvement in quality of life. There were no intraoperative complications. One patient underwent sling excision due to persistent voiding dysfunction and another patient underwent sling removal due to infection.

Oh et al. evaluated 80 women who suffered from ISD and underwent either TOA (n = 80) or TOT (n = 47) [36]. There was no difference between the two groups regarding the cure rates (TOA group, 75.6%, vs TOT group, 72.3%). Four patients (12.1%) in the TOA group underwent release of sling tension due to urinary obstruction, whereas sling tensioning was performed in five patients (15.2%). TOA procedure allows postoperative readjustment of the sling tension for a couple of days after surgery leading to good short-term results after surgery.

Patrelli et al. performed TOA procedure in 77 women with SUI and the cure rate and satisfaction rate were 90.9 and 75.3%, respectively [37]. 46.8% of the patients were immediately adjusted, whereas 14.3% of the patients had sling adjustment during hospitalization. The authors stated that the TOA was a safe and effective procedure with high rate of patient satisfaction.

5. Adjustable minislings

5.1. Altis

The Altis® (Coloplast) is an adjustable single-incision sling made of type-1 macroporous polypropylene mesh measuring 7.75 cm [38]. It has low elasticity (7.5%), which allows the maintenance of integrity under tension and two anchors, one static and one bidirectional, that allow intraoperative tension adjustment. The procedure can be performed under general, spinal, or local anesthesia. A 1.5 cm incision is made on the vaginal mucosa at the level of the midurethra. Sharp and blunt dissection is carried through the periurethral tissue and the pubic rami are reached bilaterally. The sling and the needle are advanced behind the ischiopubic rami toward the obturator space bilaterally. The needle is then removed. After the fixation of the anchors at the 2 and 10 o'clock positions, the bladder is filled with 250 ml of saline, intraoperative cough stress test is performed and the tension adjustment suture is pulled, when necessary. The adjustment thread is then cut short and the vaginal incision is closed.

Dias et al. evaluated the efficacy and complication rate of Altis® in 52 women suffering from SUI [38]. Fifty women completed the 12-month follow-up period. The subjective and objective cure rates were 84 and 90%, respectively. One case of vaginal extrusion developed requiring surgical removal of the eroded mesh. Vaginal exposure of the adjustment thread developed in three patients and was managed conservatively. De novo urgency developed in three patients and mild dyspareunia developed in two patients. The Altis® sling was found as a safe and an effective procedure for the treatment of SUI with a short-term follow-up.

Kocjancic et al. evaluated the efficacy and safety of Altis® in 113 women suffering from SUI [39]. One hundred and one women completed the 12 months of follow-up. Ninety-one women

http://dx.doi.org/10.1163/174552512X632115

(90.1%) achieved a 50% or greater reduction in pad weight and the stress test was negative in 91 (90.1%) women at 12 months. There was a significant improvement in quality of life and patient-reported outcomes. There were no reports of mesh erosion or migration through 12 months of follow-up.

Although these two studies have shown that Altis® is an efficient procedure with minimal adverse effects, it should be noted that these two studies are limited with the short follow-up period of 12 months and no randomized comparison of the procedure to other sling operations.

5.2. Ajust

Ajust™ (adjustable single-incision transobturator sling, C.R. Bard Inc., New Providence, NJ, USA) is an adjustable single-incision sling with a 1.2 cm wide macroporous polypropylene mesh. The Ajust differs from the other single-incision slings in that it has a pulley-like system that allows adjustment following insertion. The Ajust™ system consists of a curved introducer with an anchor release lever, the sling implant, one fixed anchor, one adjustable anchor, adjustment mesh, sling lock, adjusting tab and a flexible stylet (**Figure 5**).

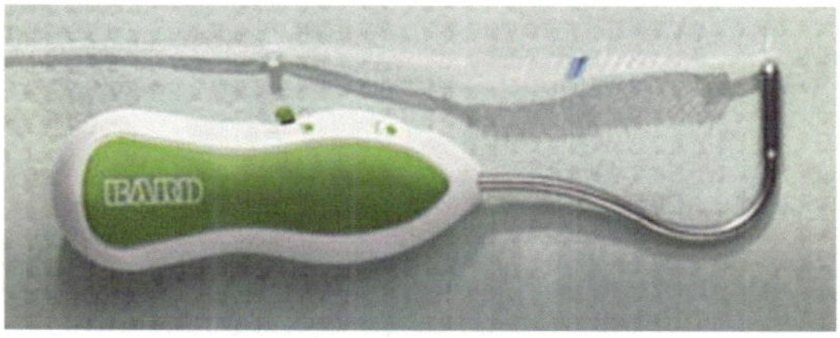

Figure 5. Ajust™ system. The sling and the curved introducer [41].

A vertical vaginal incision is performed at the level of the midurethra. Bilateral paraurethral tunnels are formed until the posterior margin of the inferior pubic rami without perforating the obturator membrane. Curved introducers loaded with self-fixating anchors are used to turn around the ischiopubic rami and fixate the anchors to obturator internus muscle and obturator membrane. Following the insertion of both anchors, the sling is adjusted in its final position by the sling lock and flexible stylet. The tension of the sling is adjusted so that the mesh is positioned in direct contact with the urethra as opposed to other retropubic or transobturator slings. Then, the adjustment mesh is cut and the vaginal incision is sutured.

In a cadaveric study, the fixation site of the anchor of the Ajust™ was studied [40]. Correct placement in the obturator membrane was achieved in 65.6% of cases. In 87.5% of cases, the anchor was placed within the complex of the obturator membrane and obturator muscles. There was more than 2 cm distance to the obturator bundle in all cases.

Meschia et al. evaluated the short-term outcomes of Ajust™ in 102 women with SUI [41]. No intraoperative complications occurred, except for technical difficulty with the fixation of the adjusting anchor on the left side of the patient. Insertion of a new Ajust tape or a TOT tape was necessary in four and two subjects, respectively. One woman suffered from urinary retention and required sling excision 9 days after surgery. The subjective and objective cure rates were 85 and 91%, respectively. There was a significant improvement in quality of life.

Similarly, Liapis et al. reported a 90% objective success rate at 6 months in 42 cases under epidural anesthesia [42]. Lucente et al., in their study, showed 91% subjective and objective success rates at 8 months in 43 women who underwent Ajust under local anesthesia [43].

Abdel-Fattah et al. evaluated the results of the Ajust™ operation with a 1-year follow-up [44]. Ninety women were operated and all completed the follow-up. Last 45 women were operated under local anesthesia. No complications occurred. Significantly, lower rates of blood loss and voiding difficulties were observed in the local anesthesia group. Subjective cure rate was 80% at the end of 1-year follow-up, with an additional 6% reporting improvement. In 13 women (14%), the procedure failed; eight reported being the same/worse and five underwent repeat surgery.

Naumann et al. compared the sexual function and quality of life following TVT and Ajust™ with a 6-month follow-up [45]. Seventy-five women underwent TVT and 75 women underwent Ajust™. Eighty-four percent of women in the Ajust™ group were cured and 9.3% were improved at the 6-month follow-up, whereas 88% of the women were cured and 6.7% were improved in the TVT group. There was a significant improvement in sexual functions and quality of life in both groups with no significant difference.

Grigoriadis et al. compared the efficacy and complication rate of Ajust™ and tension-free vaginal tape-obturator (TVT-O) [46]. The mean follow-up period was 22 months. No major intraoperative complications developed. For the TVT-O group, the objective cure rate was 86%, the improvement rate was 5.9% and the failure rate was 8.1%, while the subjective cure rate was 82.6%. For the Ajust™ group, the objective cure rate was 84.7%, the improvement rate was 4.7%, the failure rate was 10.6% and the subjective cure rate was 81.2%. Similarly, Boyers et al. compared Ajust™ with TVT-O in a total of 137 women [47]. Sixty-nine women underwent Ajust™ and 68 women underwent TVT-O. There were no significant differences between the two groups regarding subjective cure rates and improvement in quality of life. However, Ajust™ was found more cost-effective when compared to TVT-O.

Xin et al. randomized 368 women with SUI to Ajust™ or TVT-O [48]. There were no significant differences in the subjective and objective cure rates (94.4% vs 90.7% and 97.2% vs 90.7%, respectively) between Ajust™ and TVT-O. Compared with the TVT-O group, patients in the Ajust™ group had significantly less postoperative pain, shorter operative time, less intraoperative blood loss and shorter recovery time. There was no significant difference in the perioperative complications between the two groups.

Natale et al. evaluated the long-term results of Ajust™ operation [49]. Ninety-two patients completed the 2-year follow-up. The objective cure rate was 83.7% and the subjective cure rate was 81.5%. There was a significant improvement in quality of life. De novo urgency developed in nine women (9.8%). No intraoperative complications developed. Postoperative complications were leg pain in one woman, mesh extrusions in three women and recurrent urinary tract infections in one woman.

http://dx.doi.org/10.1163/174552512X632115

The main advantages of Ajust™ are its minimally invasive nature and adjustability. In a meta-analysis evaluating studies that compared single-incision slings with transobturator tape operations, similar subjective and objective cure rates were obtained and intraoperative complications were rare [50]. However, studies with long-term follow-up are needed.

6. Conclusion

Recurrent SUI and voiding dysfunction are the main problems encountered after midurethral sling operation. Adjustable midurethral slings may be used in order to avoid these problems. Some of the adjustable sling can only be adjusted during the procedure, whereas some could be adjusted at any desired time. This could prevent the requirement of additional sling surgery in patients with recurrent SUI.

There are various options of adjustable slings according to the surgical route such as retropubic or transobturator or single-incision slings or type of mesh used. Although there are studies suggesting high objective and subjective cure rates with these slings, still prospective randomized trials with long-term follow-up data are needed.

Author details

Funda Gungor Ugurlucan* and Cenk Yasa

*Address all correspondence to: fgungor@yahoo.com

Department of Obstetrics and Gynecology, Istanbul Faculty of Medicine, Istanbul University, Istanbul, Turkey

References

[1] Luber KM. The definition, prevalence and risk factors for stress urinary incontinence. Rev Urol 2004; 6(Suppl 3): S3-S9.

[2] Haylen BT, de Ridder D, Freeman RM, Swift SE, Berghmans B, Lee J, et al. An international Urogynecological Association (IUGA)/International Continence Society (ICS) joint report on the terminology for female pelvic floor dysfunction. Neurourol Urodyn 2009; 29: 4-20.

[3] Abrams P, Cardozo L, Fall M, Griffiths D, Rosier P, Ulmsten U, et al. The standardisation of terminology in lower urinary tract function: report from the standardisation subcomittee of the International Continence Society. Urology 2003; 61: 37-49.

[4] Petros PE and Ulmsten UI. An integral theory of female urinary incontinence: experimental and clinical considerations. Acta Obstet Gynecol Scand 1997; 166(Suppl): 3-8.

[5] Ulmsten U, Henriksson L, Johnson P, Varhos G. An ambulatory surgical procedure under local anaesthesia for treatment of female urinary incontinence. Int Urogynecol J 1996; 7:81-86.

[6] Delorme E. Transobturator urethral suspension: mini-invasive procedure in the treatment of stress urinary incontinence in women. Prog Urol 2001; 6:1306-1313.

[7] Abdel-Fattah M, Ford JA, Lim CP, Madhuvrata P. Single-incision mini-slings versus standard midurethral slings in surgical management of female stress urinary incontinence: a meta-analysis of effectiveness and complications. Eur Urol 2011; 60: 468-480.

[8] Ford AA, Rogerson L, Cody JD, Ogah J. Mid-urethral sling operations for stress urinary incontinence in women. Cochrane Database Syst Rev 2015; (7): CD006375.

[9] Nilsson CG, Palva K, Pezapour M, Falconer C. Eleven years prospective follow-up of the tension-free vaginal tape procedure for treatment of stress urinary incontinence. Int Urogynecol J Pelvic Floor Dysfunct 2008; 19: 1043-1047.

[10] Schimpf MO, Rahn DD, Wheeler TL, Patel M, White AB, Orejuela FJ, et al. Sling surgery for stress urinary incontinence in women: a systematic review and metaanalysis. Am J Obstet Gynecol 2014; 211: 71.e1-71.e27.

[11] Liapis A, Bakas P, Creatsas G. Tension-free vaginal tape in the management of recurrent urodynamic stress incontinence after previous failed midurethral tape. Eur Urol 2009; 55: 1450-1455.

[12] Jonsson Funk M, Siddiqui NY, Kawasaki A, Wu JM. Long-term outcomes after stress urinary incontinence surgery. Obstet Gynecol 2012; 120: 83-90.

[13] Iglesias X, Espuna M. Surgical treatment of urinary stress incontinence using a method for postoperative adjustment of sling tension. Int Urogynecol J Pelvic Floor Dysfunct 2003; 14: 326-330.

[14] Mantovani F, Castelnuovo C, Bernardini P. ReMeEx device (External Mechanic Regulator) for incontinence implantation and regulation procedure, complications and results at 3 years follow-up. Arch Ital Urol Androl 2004; 76: 49-50.

[15] Yoo DH, Noh JH. Readjustable sling procedure for the treatment of female stress urinary incontinence with intrinsic sphincter deficiency: preliminary report. Korean J Urol 2010;51:420-425.

[16] Araco F, Gravante G, Dati S, Bulzomi' V, Sesti F, Piccione E. Results 1 year after the Reemex system was applied for the treatment of stress urinary incontinence caused by intrinsic sphincter deficiency. Int Urogynecol J Pelvic Floor Dysfunct 2008;19:783-786.

[17] Moreno Sierra J, Marques Queimadelos A, Arano Beltran P, De La Fuente Perez P, Cerezela Requena JF, Cortes Otero E, et al. Spanish registry of TRT Reemex system in women with stress urinary incontinence (SUI). Arch Esp Urol 2006; 59: 169-174.

[18] Errando C, Rodriguez-Escovar F, Gutierrez C, Baez C, Arano P, Villavicencio H. A re-adjustable sling for female recurrent stress incontinence and sphincteric deficiency: outcomes and complications in 125 patients using the Remeex Sling System. Neurourol Urodyn 2010; 29: 1429-1432.

[19] Park BH, Kim JC, Kim HW, Kim YH, Choi JB, Lee DH. Midterm efficacy and complications of Readjustable Midurethral Sling (Remeex System) in female stress urinary incontinence with recurrence or intrinsic sphincter deficiency. Urology 2015; 85: 79-84.

[20] Yasa C, Gungor Ugurlucan F, Dural O, Celik S, Yalcın O. A valuable option in the management of female recurrent stress urinary incontinence: re-adjustable sling (Remeex Sling System). Urol Int. 2016;97(2):224-9.

[21] Barrington J, Archer R, Kulkarni M, Forrest A. The TRT Female Remeex System for recurrent female stress urinary incontinence: a 5-year follow-up study. J Obstet Gynaecol 2013; 33: 391-393.

[22] Giberti C, Gallo F, Cortese P, Schenone M. The suburethral tension adjustable sling (Remeex system) in the treatment of female urinary incontinence due to 'true' intrinsic sphincter deficiency: results after 5 years of mean follow-up. BJU Int 2011; 108: 1140-1144.

[23] Lorenzo-Gómez MF, Padilla-Fernández B, Virseda-Rodríguez AJ, Collazos-Robles RE, García-Cenador MB, Mirón-Canelo JA. Severe complications and failures of incontinence surgery using the Remeex(®) adjustable tension sling (external mechanical regulator) Actas Urol Esp 2015; 39(9): 558-563. doi: 10.1016/j.acuro.2015.05.001.

[24] Romero Maroto J, Ortiz Gorraiz MO, Prieto Chaparro L, Pacheco Bru JJ, Mirales Bueno JJ, Lopez Lopez C. Transvaginal adjustable tape: an adjustable mesh for surgical treatment of female stress urinary incontinence. Int Urogynecol J Pelvic Floor Dysfunct 2008; 19: 1109-1116.

[25] Kuschel S, Schuessler B. Results on function and safety of the Safyre-t a hybrid transobturator vaginal sling for the treatment of stress urinary incontinence. Neurourol Urodyn 2008; 27: 403-406.

[26] Palma PCR, Riccetto CLZ, Dambros M. SAFYRE: a readjustable minimally invasive sling for female urinary stress incontinence. Int Braz J Urol 2003; 29(4):353-359.

[27] Palma PCR, Dambros M, Riccetto CZ, Thiel M, Netto NR. The Ibero-American experience with a re-adjustable minimally invasive sling. BJU Int 2004; 95: 341-345.

[28] Palma PCR, Riccetto CLZ, Dambros M, Thiel M. Safyre sling: early results of a new tension-adjustable and self anchoring device for female stress incontinence. J Endourol 2002; 16(Suppl 1): Abst P25–2.

[29] Palma P, Riccetto C, Herrmann V, Dambros M, Thiel M, Bandiera S, Netto NR Jr. Transobturator SAFYRE sling is as effective as the transvaginal procedure. Int Urogynecol J Pelvic Floor Dysfunct 2005; 16(6): 487-491.

[30] Silva-Filho AL, Candido EB, Noronha A, Triginelli SA. Comparative study of autologous pubovaginal sling and synthetic transobturator (TOT) Safyre sling in the treatment of stress urinary incontinence. Arch Gynecol Obstet 2006; 273: 288-292.

[31] Govier FE, Kobashi KC, Kozlowski PM, et al. High complication rate identified in sacrocolpopexy patients attributed to silicone mesh. Urology 2005; 65: 1099-1103.

[32] Duckett JR, Constantine G. Complications of silicone sling insertion for stress urinary incontinence. J Urol 2000; 163: 1835-1837.

[33] Yamada BS, Govier FE, Stefanovic KB, et al. High rate of vaginal erosions associated with the mentor ObTape. J Urol 2006; 176: 651-654.

[34] Padilla-Fernández B, Begoña García-Cenador M, Gómez-García A, Mirón-Canelo JA, Gil-Vicente A, Silva-Abuín JM, Lorenzo-Gómez MF. Results of the surgical correction of urinary stress incontinence according to the type of transobturator tape utilized. Archives of Italian Urology and Andrology 2013; 85(3): 149-153.

[35] Lee SY, Lee YS, Lee HN, Choo MS, Lee JG, Kim HG, Woo JK, Lee KS. Transobturator adjustable tape for severe stress urinary incontinence and stress urinary incontinence with voiding dysfunction. Int Urogynecol J 2011; 22: 341-346.

[36] Oh TH, Shin JH, Na YG. A comparison of the clinical efficacy of the transobturator adjustable tape (TOA) and transobturator tape (TOT) for treating female stress urinary incontinence with intrinsic sphincter deficiency: short-term results. Korean J Urol 2012; 53: 98-103.

[37] Patrelli TS, Gizzo S, Noventa M, Dall'Asta A, Musaro A, Faioli R, et al. Female stress urinary incontinence: clinical efficacy and satisfaction after transobturator adjustable tape sling: an observational longitudinal cohort study. Surg Innov 2015; 22: 137-142.

[38] Dias J, Xambre L, Costa L, Costa P, Ferraz L. Short-term outcomes of Altis single-incision procedure for stress urinary incontinence: a prospective single-center study. Int Urogynecol J 2014; 25: 1089-1095.

[39] Kocjancic E, Tu L, Erickson T, Gheiler E, Drie DV. The safety and efficacy of a new adjustable single incision sling for female stress urinary incontinence. J Urol 2014; 192: 1477-1482.

[40] Hubka P, Nanka O, Martan A, Svabik K, El-Haddad R, Masata J. Fixation of the Ajust minisling based upon cadaveric study. Int Urogynecol J 2013; 24: 2119- 2123.

[41] Meschia M, Barbacini P, Baccichet R, Buanoguidi A, Maffiolini M, Ricci L, Braghin C, Brusati V, Dell'Utri C, Spreafico L. Short-term outcomes with the Ajust™ system: a new single incision sling for the treatment of stress urinary incontinence. Int Urogynecol J 2011; 22: 177-182.

[42] Liapis A, Georgantopoulou C, Bakas P, et al. Short term results of the Ajust adjustable single incision sling procedure for the treatment of urodynamic stress urinary incontinence. Int J Urogynaecol 2010; 2(Suppl 1): 778.

http://dx.doi.org/10.1163/174552512X632115

[43] Lucente V , Cornu J , Sèbe P , Peyrat L, Ciofu C, Haab F. Ajust single incision transobturator sling procedure for stress urinary incontinence in women: one year results. Int J Urogynaecol 2010; 2(Suppl 1): 775.

[44] Abdel-Fattah M, Agur W, Abdel-All M, Guerrero K, Allam M, Mackintosh A, et al. Prospective multi-centre study of adjustable single-incision mini-sling (Ajust) in the management of stress urinary incontinence in women: 1-year follow-up study. BJU Int 2012; 109: 880-886.

[45] Naumann G, Hagemeier T, Zachmann S, Aktham A, Albrich S, Skala C, et al. Long-term outcomes of the Ajust adjustable single-incision sling fort he treatment of stress urinary incontinence. Int Urogynecol J 2013; 24: 231-239.

[46] Grigoriadis C, Bakas P, Derpapas A, Creatsa M, Liapis A. Tension-free vaginal tape-obturator versus Ajust adjustable single incision sling procedure in women with urodynamic stress urinary incontinence. Eur J Obstet Gynecol Reprod Biol 2013; 170: 563-566.

[47] Boyers D, Kilonzo M, Mostafa A, Abdel-Fattah M. Comparison of an adjustable anchored single-incision minisling, Ajust®, with a standard midurethral sling, TVT-O™: a health economic evaluation. BJU Int 2013; 112: 1169-1177.

[48] Xin X, Song Y, Xia Z. A comparison between adjustable single-incision sling and tension-free vaginal tape-obturator in treating stress urinary incontinence. Arch Gynecol Obstet 2016; 293: 457-463.

[49] Natale F, Dati S, La Penna C, Rombola P, Capello S, Piccione E. Single incision sling (Ajust) for the treatment of female stress urinary incontinence: 2 year follow-up. Eur J Obstet Gynecol Reprod Biol 2014; 182: 48-52.

[50] Zhang P, Fan B, Zhang P, Han H, Xu Y, Wang B, et al. Meta-analysis of female stress urinary incontinence treatments with adjustable single incision minislings and transobturator tension-free vaginal tape surgeries. BMC Urol 2015; 15: 64.

Section 3

Conservative Treatment

Chapter 3

Complementary and Alternative Medicine Treatment for Urinary Incontinence

Ran Pang, Ri Chang, Xin-Yao Zhou and
Chun-Lan Jin

Additional information is available at the end of the chapter

http://dx.doi.org/10.5772/66705

Abstract

Complementary and alternative medicine has been widely used for various diseases and gained acceptance throughout the industrialized world. Basically, complementary and alternative medicine is grouped into five domains: biologically based therapies, mind-body interventions, manipulative and body-based approaches, energy therapies and whole medical systems. Each domain covers a number of therapies. In this chapter, we present the evidence about effectiveness of each complementary and alternative medicine therapy as well as the possible mechanism on the treatment of urinary incontinence. Besides reviewing existed evidence, our research and clinical experience are also presented.

Keywords: urinary incontinence, complementary and alternative medicine, acupuncture

1. Introduction

Urinary incontinence (UI) is common in adult population. It is estimated that about half of women suffer from UI [1]. In men, UI mainly occurs secondary to prostatectomy. The reported prevalence of UI following radical prostatectomy is as high as 50% [2]. In general, UI is classified into stress urinary incontinence (SUI), urgency urinary incontinence (UUI), mixed urinary incontinence (MUI) and overflow urinary incontinence (OUI). Although a number of treatments are available for different types of UI, some patients still cannot get benefit from these therapeutic measures. Furthermore, adverse events related to the treatment bother both patients and their doctors. For these reasons, plenty of patients resort to complementary and alternative medicine (CAM) therapies. In this chapter, we present the evidence for the efficacy of CAM on different types of UI.

CAM refers to a series of medical and health care practices and products that are not considered to be part of conventional medicine [3]. The National Center for Complementary and Alternative Medicine at the National Institutes of Health (NIH) has grouped CAM into five domains: (1) biologically based therapies, such as dietary modifications and nutraceuticals; (2) mind-body interventions, such as biofeedback and yoga; (3) manipulative and body-based approaches, such as massage; (4) energy therapies, such as Qigong and Reiki; (5) whole medical systems, such as traditional Chinese medicine, acupuncture and naturopathy [4].

2. Biologically based therapies

2.1. Dietary modifications

It is reported that some food and beverages may aggravate UI. Of those, caffeinated beverages are considered to play an important role in inducing UI due to their diuretic effect. A prospective cohort study of more than 65,000 women found that excessive caffeine intake (≥450 mg/day) was associated with an increased incidence of UI [5]. A case-control study demonstrated that high caffeine intake (≥400 mg/day) might cause detrusor overactivity which is related to UUI based on urodynamic evaluation [6]. A recent cross-sectional study, US National Health and Nutrition Examination Survey, further revealed that moderate caffeine intake (≥204 mg/day) was associated with UI in female population [7]. Based on these finding, some studies were designed to identify the efficacy of caffeine reduction on improvement of UI symptoms. Tomlinson et al. found that UI patients could get significant benefit from a caffeine reduction education. In this study, 41 patients' daily caffeinated beverages consumption was reduced from 829 ± 385 to 489 ± 312 ml in 4 weeks. As a result, their daily urinary leakage and UI episode were decreased from 42.21 ± 77.34 to 24.09 ± 40.93 and from 2.60 ± 2.65 to 1.68 ± 1.52, respectively [8]. By contrast, outcomes from a prospective randomized trial showed that reduced caffeine intake could only improve patients' symptoms of frequency and urgency significantly, but had no effect on reduction of urinary leakage [9]. A prospective cohort study further revealed that caffeine reduction could not decrease the risk of UI progression over 2 years [10].

Besides caffeinated beverages, carbonated drinks are considered as another daily consumption which may exacerbate the UI symptoms. In a prospective cohort study, the lower urinary tract symptoms (LUTS), diet and lifestyle from 7046 women were collected and analyzed. It confirmed that consumption of carbonated drinks was a significant risk factor for occurrence of SUI [11]. Another study found that only excessive consumption of carbonated beverages was associated with the increased risk of UI [12]. Additionally, Thomas and his colleague found that some other diets and beverages including spicy foods, citrus juices and tomato-based products could trigger UI [13]. On the contrary, outcomes from a large prospective cohort study demonstrated that citrus juice consumption decreased the risk of storage LUTS progression in men [14].

Whether fluid intake should be restricted in UI patients is another issue. Swithinbank et al. performed a randomized, prospective, crossover study to assess the effect of increasing and decreasing fluid intake on symptoms in women with UUI or SUI. They found that fluid intake restriction could decrease the episode of both UUI and SUI significantly [15]. Another study, however, showed that increased fluid intake was not related to episode of UI; even an increased urine volume was observed [8]. Hashim et al. further explored the relationship

http://dx.doi.org/10.5772/66705

between fluid intake restriction and LUTS in patients with overactive bladder (OAB). They found that a 25% reduction in fluid intake could relieve OAB symptoms, but not UI [16].

Despite inconsistent evidence, a dietary modification to decrease intake of fluid, caffeine and carbonated drinks is recommended for all UI patients [17]. On the other hand, an individuated strategy in dietary change should be taken into consideration for each patient. We advise patients to eliminate all the foods and beverages which may worsen UI from their diet for at least 1 week. Then the comestibles will be added one by one to identify the sensitive foods and beverages. After that, an individuated dietary modification strategy can be established and practiced. The reported foods and beverages with potential negative effect for UI patients are listed in **Table 1**.

Category	Specific items
Beverages	Coffee (caffeinated and decaffeinated)
	Tea (caffeinated)
	Carbonated beverages(cola, non-cola, diet, and caffeine-free)
	Alcoholic drinks (liquor, beer, wine and champagne)
Fruits and vegetables	Citrus juice
	Tomato and tomato products
Other foods	Spicy foods

Table 1. Foods and beverages affecting UI.

3. Mind-body interventions

3.1. Pelvic floor muscle training

Pelvic floor muscle training (PFMT) is a common regimen for patients with UI. On one hand, it can improve SUI by increasing pelvic floor muscle tone. On the other hand, contraction of pelvic floor muscle induced by PFMT inhibits detrusor overactivity, which can reduce the episode of UUI. In a randomized, controlled trial, 130 female patients with SUI or MUI were allocated into PFMT or control group. After 12 weeks treatment, the average leakage assessed by 1-h pad test dropped from 5.1 to 1.5 g significantly in PFMT group, whereas the counterpart increased from 4.6 to 5.1 g in control group. Additionally, pelvic floor muscle strength was increased markedly in PFMT group, while not in control group [18]. A systematic review published in Cochrane collaboration has further confirmed the efficacy of PFMT for SUI, UUI and MUI [19]. That review also revealed that the effect of PFMT on MUI is lower than the one on pure SUI. In terms of PFMT procedure, patients normally are asked to squeeze the muscles which they use to stop the urine flow. Once they can identify the right muscles, they need to hold the contraction for 5 s and then relax for 5 s. To obtain substantial benefit, PFMT program should comprise at least eight pelvic floor muscle contractions performed three times per day. With regard to the duration, PFMT is recommended to be performed for at least 8–12 weeks. Unfortunately, the majority of patients with UI fail to practice a long-term PFMT. In a follow-up study, Beyar and his colleague found that the rate of 5-year adherence to PFMT in women with SUI was only 41.6% [20]. Another early study showed that only 28% of patients adhered to practice PFMT during the 15-year follow-up period [21].

3.2. Bladder training

Bladder training is a self-control technique suppressing urge to urinate, which can reduce the episode of UUI. The common technique of bladder training is timed voiding. To practice timed voiding, patients need to complete a 3-day bladder diary first. Based on the diary, the interval between two micturations is easy to determine. Then a voiding schedule can be drawn up by adding about 15 min to the voiding interval. Patients are asked to comply with the voiding schedule, no matter whether they actually feel the urge to void. Once patients are accustomed to the current schedule, the amount of time between micturations will be increased gradually, until they can last for 3 h without having to go to the bathroom. Traditionally, bladder training is used for treatment of UUI. Some studies found that bladder training was also effective for SUI and MUI. A systematic review has demonstrated the efficacy of bladder training on UUI, SUI and MUI [22]. A randomized controlled trial compared the effects of bladder training and PFMT on SUI in elderly women. The result showed that bladder training is less effective than PFMT in management of SUI [23]. It is noteworthy that bladder training needs to be performed at least 6 weeks in order to achieve a satisfactory benefit. In addition, patients may experience a significant discomfort during bladder training. To ensure patients can accept the therapy, they should be sufficiently educated prior to bladder training.

3.3. Biofeedback

Biofeedback, as a technique enhancing the effect of PFMT, typically uses a device to record the biological signals when patients contract their pelvic floor muscle voluntarily and present the information to patients, which can help patients to perform the right PFMT. A systematic review showed that biofeedback could provide benefit in addition to PFMT for women with SUI, UUI and MUI [24]. However, a later randomized, controlled study revealed that biofeedback had no add-on effect in women with SUI compared to PFMT alone [25]. A study showed that 55% of patients with UUI achieved an improvement of more than 50%. That study also found that patients with severe detrusor overactivity had poor response to biofeedback [26]. According to our experience, biofeedback is more effective for women with pure SUI than counterparts with UUI or MUI. Besides SUI, UUI and MUI, we also find that biofeedback may be helpful for patients with OUI, although they normally need catheterization or other invasive treatment. The possible reason might result from the urethral muscle relaxation induced by biofeedback.

3.4. Yoga

Yoga, a series of exercises originated in ancient India, can regulate the physical and mental function spontaneously. It is reported that yoga can modulate pelvic floor muscle tone, which contributes to LUTS relief [27]. A study showed that yoga could improve the symptoms of UUI and enhance the quality of life [28]. In a randomized, controlled trial, 19 women with SUI, UUI or MUI were allocated to yoga therapy or control group. After 6-week therapy, women in yoga therapy group presented a more significant decrease in daily episode of UI than counterparts in control group (1.8 vs. 0.3) [29]. In terms of specific yoga postures, frog pose, fish pose, locust pose, plank pose, sitting forward bend and seated twist may be beneficial for UI [27].

http://dx.doi.org/10.5772/66705

4. Manipulative and body-based approaches

4.1. Massage

Massage refers to a series of actions on the body with appropriate pressure to make muscle relaxed. Kassolik et al. tried to treat a 50-year-old woman with SUI using massage. Following 4 weeks treatment, the patient reported a 100% improvement on her SUI [30]. Although only limited evidence is available, we find that massage is effective for SUI, UUI and MUI. Based on our clinical experience, the majority of patients can get benefits from six to eight sessions of massage focusing on the pelvic floor muscles. The possible mechanism includes the relaxation of pelvic floor muscle induced by massage and regulation effect of massage on central nervous system [31].

5. Energy therapies

It has been widely accepted that energy therapies are helpful for people to maintain their health. A retrospective study reviewed the effect of extracorporeal magnetic energy stimulation on symptoms in women with SUI and OAB. In that study, 72 patients completed a 9-week therapy of magnetic energy stimulation. After treatment, the majority of patients achieved a significant improvement in their symptoms [32]. Qigong, as an important component of energy therapies, has been used to treat many chronic diseases. However, there have not been substantial evidence for its effectiveness on UI. Despite the lack of evidence, we find that Qigong can improve the symptoms in some patients with SUI, UUI or MUI according to our clinical experience. However, the efficacy of Qigong usually varies and depends on an individual's confidence for this energy therapy.

6. Whole medical systems

6.1. Acupuncture

Acupuncture, as an effective therapy, has gained acceptance in urologists over the past decades [33]. A number of studies have shown its efficacy on different types of UI. In order to present the evidence in a clear way, we discuss the effect of acupuncture on SUI, UUI, MUI and OUI, respectively.

6.1.1. SUI

Although many studies have reported the efficacy of acupuncture on SUI, most of them are retrospective and only with a small sample size, which causes the results controversial. Moreover, lack of appropriate control is a main issue in clinical trial of acupuncture. To overcome these limitation, we designed several single-blind, randomized, controlled trails. More importantly, we created a new pragmatic placebo needle, which has been confirmed to be able to achieve blindness for patients in clinical trials. In terms of the specific procedure, a small pad is adhered to patients' skin of each acupoint before performing acupuncture. A blunt needle is used to pierce the pad without penetrating the skin in control group, while a normal needle penetrates the skin through the pad [34]. In phase I clinical trial, a total of 70 patients with SUI were allocated to receiving electro-acupuncture or placebo electro-acupuncture three time a week for 3 weeks. The selected acupoints included bilateral BL33 (Zhong Liao) located in the third sacral foramen and BL35 (Hui Yang) lateral to the tip of the coccyx. In acupuncture group, normal needles were inserted with a depth of 50 mm. After a De Qi sensation was obtained, paired electrodes of electro-acupuncture apparatus were attached transversely to bilateral BL33 and BL35, respectively, with a continuous wave (50 Hz) for 30 min, three times a week. By contrast, the placebo needles were used at same acupoints and the same parameters of electro-acupuncture device were used in control group. Based on the study design, each patient was asked to complete 1-h pad test, 3 days bladder diary and the International Consultation on Incontinence questionnaire short form (ICIQ-SF) at baseline and posttreatment to assess the effectiveness of acupuncture. After 6-week treatment, the urine leakage evaluated by 1-h pad test was reduced more significantly in electro-acupuncture group in comparison with counterparts in control group (2.3 g vs. 0.3 g), so did the episodes of SUI (2.0 vs. 0.7). Moreover, a significant decrease in ICIQ-SF score was found in electro-acupuncture group compared to control group after treatment, which means that patients in electro-acupuncture group gained a more improvement in SUI symptoms [35].

To further assess the long-term effect of acupuncture, a multicentered, randomized, controlled, phase II trial was designed. In this ongoing study, patients will be followed as long as 24 weeks after they receive 18 sessions of electro-acupuncture therapy [36]. In addition, another randomized, controlled trial is also ongoing, in which the effect of electro-acupuncture is compared with the PFMT [37]. We hope that the results of these clinical trials can bring us sufficient evidence for the effect of acupuncture on SUI.

6.1.2. UUI

Although anticholinergics have been considered as the first-line drug for OAB and UUI, as high as 30–50% of patients cannot get benefit from the pharmacological therapy [38]. A single-blind, randomized, controlled study investigated the effect of acupuncutre on OAB refractory to anticholinergics. In it, 50 patients with OAB who had poor response to anticholinergics were given electro-acupuncuture or sham electro-acupuncuture randomly for 6 weeks. Based on the procedure, needles were inserted into bilateral BL32 (Ci Liao) located in the secondary foramen, BL33 and BL34 (Xia Liao) located in the fourth foramen at an angle of 60° horizontal and 30° sagittal with a depth of about 50 mm and each pair of needles were connected to electro-acupuncture device, with a disperse-dense (4/20 Hz) wave for 30 min, five sessions a week in electro-acupuncture group. By contrast, non-acupoints with superficial needles were used as control intervention. To assess the effect of acupuncture objectively, urodynamics were used to measure patients' bladder function at baseline and posttreatment. After 6-week treatment, a significant improvement in the first sensation of bladder filling, first urge to void and maximum cystometric capacity were observed in electro-acupuncture group, while no change in control group [39]. In another randomized, controlled trail, 199 patients with UUI were assigned into electro-acupuncture or pharmacological therapy group with a ratio of 2:1. For patients in electro-acupuncture group, two groups of acupoints were selected to perform acupuncture alternately. One included

CV3 (Zhong Ji) located in the midline and above the pubic symphysis, bilateral KI12 (Da He) which is lateral to CV3, ST28 (Shui Dao) which is lateral to the midline and below the navel, and SP6 (San Yin Jiao) situated above the tip of the medial malleolus on the posterior border of the tibia. Of those, KI12 and ST28 were connected to the electrodes of electro-acupuncture equipment with a disperse-dense (4/20 Hz) wave for 30 min, three sessions a week. Another one includes bilateral BL32, BL35, BL29 (Zhong Lv Shu) located lateral to the midline and at the height of the third sacral foramen, and BL40 (Wei Zhong) situated in the midpoint of transverse crease of popliteal fossa. Of those, BL32 and BL35 were connected to a pair of wires of electro-acupuncture apparatus with the same parameters of electro-acupuncture device. As the control, patients in pharmacological group received oral tolterodine 2 mg, twice a day. After 3-week treatment, the ICIQ-SF score in electro-acupuncture group dropped from 4.06 ± 1.36 to 1.57 ± 1.14 ($P < 0.01$), while no significant difference was found in pharmacological therapy group [40].

6.1.3. MUI

MUI is a complicated disorder involving bladder and urethral function. Patients with MUI normally have poor response to both pharmacological and surgical treatment. To determine the effect of acupuncture on MUI, we designed a pilot study. In it, 42 women with MUI received acupuncture therapy for 8 weeks. The selected acupoints include bilateral BL32, BL35, SP6 and ST36 (Zu San Li) located below the lower border of the patella and lateral to the anterior border of the tibia. Of those, BL32 and BL35 were connected to the electrodes of electro-acupuncture equipment with a disperse-dense (4/20 Hz) wave for 30 min, three sessions a week. After 8-week treatment, the majority of patients presented a significant decrease in ICIQ-SF score and the episode of UI, so did the daily urine leakage [41].

We further designed a randomized, controlled trail to explore the synergy effect of acupuncture and anticholinergics. In this trial, 71 patients with MUI were allocated to combination therapy group or acupuncture group. Patients in each group received acupuncture therapy with same procedure in the pilot study and ones in combination therapy group received additional tolterodine 2 mg orally twice a day. After 8 weeks treatment, patients in combination therapy group presented a more significant reduction in daily urine leakage than the counterparts in control group, although no marked difference was found in cured and response rate between two groups [42].

6.1.4. OUI

Patients with OUI usually need to be treated with catheterization or invasive therapy. There have not been studies focusing on the effect of acupuncture in treating OUI so far. We designed a prospective, randomized, controlled trial to investigate the effect of acupuncture in preventing bladder over-distension, an important reason of OUI. In it, 61 patients underwent spinal anesthesia were allocated to receiving acupuncture or no intervention. Based on the procedure, acupuncture was performed when patients' sensory level regressed to T10 segment during anesthesia. The selected acupoints included CV3, CV4 (Guan Yuan) located below CV3 and bilateral ST29 (Gui Lai) situated below the navel and lateral to the midline. After the needles were inserted in these points with a depth of approximately 25 mm, the handles of needles were connected to electrodes of nerve stimulator with a low-frequency (2 Hz) continuous wave for 30 min. The incidence of bladder over-distentsion and urinary retention, the time to voluntary micturition after spinal anesthesia, urine volume and adverse events were collected and compared between two groups to evaluate the effect of acupuncture. During post-anesthesia follow-up, a significant lower incidence of bladder over-distension (16.1% vs. 53.3%, $P < 0.01$) and shorter time to voluntary micturition (228 ± 78 min vs. 313 ± 91 min, $P < 0.01$) were found in acupuncture group compared to control group. By contrast, no marked differences were detected in incidence of urinary retention, urinary volume and side effects between two groups [43]. Because the findings of this study suggest that acupuncture can decrease the incidence of bladder over-distension in patients undergoing spinal anesthesia, it might be reasonable to infer that acupuncture is effective for treatment of OUI. However, the exact effect of acupuncture on OUI needs to be confirmed by well-designed clinical trial.

7. Summary

There have been increasing evidence on effectiveness of CAM therapies for different types of UI. However, the majority of studies have non-blind design and small sample size, which limits the level of evidence. Despite these limitations, CAM therapies should be considered as the initial management for patient with UI since they are relatively noninvasive and can benefit a substantial group of UI patients.

Acknowledgements

This work was supported by Beijing Municipal Science & Technology Commission No. Z161100000516156 and grant 2014S292 from Guang An Men Hospital, China Academy of Chinese Medical Sciences.

Author details

Ran Pang[1]*, Ri Chang[2], Xin-Yao Zhou[3] and Chun-Lan Jin[4]

*Address all correspondence to: pangran2002@gmail.com

1 Department of Urology, Guang An Men Hospital, China Academy of Chinese Medical Sciences, Beijing, PR China

2 Beijing University of Chinese Medicine, Beijing, PR China

3 Department of Internal Medicine, Guang An Men Hospital, China Academy of Chinese Medical Sciences, Beijing, PR China

4 Institute of Acupuncture and Moxibustion, China Academy of Chinese Medical Sciences, Beijing, PR China

References

[1] Minassian, V.A., W.F. Stewart, and G.C. Wood, *Urinary incontinence in women: variation in prevalence estimates and risk factors*. Obstet Gynecol, 2008. **111**(2 Pt 1): pp. 324–31.

[2] Ostrowski, I., et al., *Current interventional management of male stress urinary incontinence following urological procedures*. Cent Eur J Urol, 2015. **68**(3): pp. 340–7.

[3] Barnes, P.M., B. Bloom, and R.L. Nahin, *Complementary and alternative medicine use among adults and children: United States, 2007*. Natl Health Stat Rep, 2008. (12): pp. 1–23.

[4] Moquin, B., et al., *Complementary and alternative medicine (CAM)*. Geriatr Nurs, 2009. **30**(3): pp. 196–203.

[5] Jura, Y.H., et al., *Caffeine intake, and the risk of stress, urgency and mixed urinary incontinence*. J Urol, 2011. **185**(5): pp. 1775–80.

[6] Arya, L.A., D.L. Myers, and N.D. Jackson, *Dietary caffeine intake and the risk for detrusor instability: a case-control study*. Obstet Gynecol, 2000. **96**(1): pp. 85–9.

[7] Gleason, J.L., et al., *Caffeine and urinary incontinence in US women*. Int Urogynecol J, 2013. **24**(2): pp. 295–302.

[8] Tomlinson, B.U., et al., *Dietary caffeine, fluid intake and urinary incontinence in older rural women*. Int Urogynecol J Pelvic Floor Dysfunct, 1999. **10**(1): pp. 22–8.

[9] Bryant, C.M., C.J. Dowell, and G. Fairbrother, *Caffeine reduction education to improve urinary symptoms*. Br J Nurs, 2002. **11**(8): pp. 560–5.

[10] Townsend, M.K., N.M. Resnick, and F. Grodstein, *Caffeine intake and risk of urinary incontinence progression among women*. Obstet Gynecol, 2012. **119**(5): pp. 950–7.

[11] Dallosso, H.M., et al., *The association of diet and other lifestyle factors with overactive bladder and stress incontinence: a longitudinal study in women*. BJU Int, 2003. **92**(1): pp. 69–77.

[12] Ozgur Yeniel, A., et al., *The prevalence of probable overactive bladder, associated risk factors and its effect on quality of life among Turkish midwifery students*. Eur J Obstet Gynecol Reprod Biol, 2012. **164**(1): pp. 105–9.

[13] Thomas, A.M. and J.M. Morse, *Managing urinary incontinence with self-care practices*. J Gerontol Nurs, 1991. **17**(6): pp. 9–14.

[14] Maserejian, N.N., et al., *Intake of caffeinated, carbonated, or citrus beverage types and development of lower urinary tract symptoms in men and women*. Am J Epidemiol, 2013. **177**(12): pp. 1399–410.

[15] Swithinbank, L., H. Hashim, and P. Abrams, *The effect of fluid intake on urinary symptoms in women*. J Urol, 2005. **174**(1): pp. 187–9.

[16] Hashim, H. and P. Abrams, *How should patients with an overactive bladder manipulate their fluid intake?* BJU Int, 2008. **102**(1): pp. 62–6.

[17] Wood, L.N. and J.T. Anger, *Urinary incontinence in women*. BMJ, 2014. **349**: p. g4531.

[18] Celiker Tosun, O., et al., *Does pelvic floor muscle training abolish symptoms of urinary incontinence? A randomized controlled trial*. Clin Rehabil, 2015. **29**(6): pp. 525–37.

[19] Dumoulin, C., E.J. Hay-Smith, and G. Mac Habee-Seguin, *Pelvic floor muscle training versus no treatment, or inactive control treatments, for urinary incontinence in women*. Cochrane Database Syst Rev, 2014. (5): p. CD005654.

[20] Beyar, N. and A. Groutz, *Pelvic floor muscle training for female stress urinary incontinence: five years outcomes*. Neurourol Urodyn, 2015. [Epub ahead of print].

[21] Bo, K., B. Kvarstein, and I. Nygaard, *Lower urinary tract symptoms and pelvic floor muscle exercise adherence after 15 years*. Obstet Gynecol, 2005. **105**(5 Pt 1): pp. 999–1005.

[22] Wallace, S.A., et al., *Bladder training for urinary incontinence in adults*. Cochrane Database Syst Rev, 2004. (1): p. CD001308.

[23] Sherburn, M., et al., *Incontinence improves in older women after intensive pelvic floor muscle training: an assessor-blinded randomized controlled trial*. Neurourol Urodyn, 2011. **30**(3): pp. 317–24.

[24] Herderschee, R., et al., *Feedback or biofeedback to augment pelvic floor muscle training for urinary incontinence in women*. Cochrane Database Syst Rev, 2011. (7): p. CD009252.

[25] Hirakawa, T., et al., *Randomized controlled trial of pelvic floor muscle training with or without biofeedback for urinary incontinence*. Int Urogynecol J, 2013. **24**(8): pp. 1347–54.

[26] Resnick, N.M., et al., *What predicts and what mediates the response of urge urinary incontinence to biofeedback?* Neurourol Urodyn, 2013. **32**(5): pp. 408–15.

[27] Ripoll, E. and D. Mahowald, *Hatha Yoga therapy management of urologic disorders*. World J Urol, 2002. **20**(5): pp. 306–9.

[28] Tenfelde, S. and L.W. Janusek, *Yoga: a biobehavioral approach to reduce symptom distress in women with urge urinary incontinence*. J Altern Complement Med, 2014. **20**(10): pp. 737–42.

[29] Huang, A.J., et al., *A group-based yoga therapy intervention for urinary incontinence in women: a pilot randomized trial*. Female Pelvic Med Reconstr Surg, 2014. **20**(3): pp. 147–54.

[30] Kassolik, K., et al., *The effectiveness of massage in stress urinary incontinence-case study*. Rehabil Nurs, 2013. **38**(6): pp. 306–14.

[31] Field, T., *Massage therapy research review*. Complement Ther Clin Pract, 2014. **20**(4): pp. 224–9.

[32] Lo, T.S., et al., *Effect of extracorporeal magnetic energy stimulation on bothersome lower urinary tract symptoms and quality of life in female patients with stress urinary incontinence and overactive bladder*. J Obstet Gynaecol Res, 2013. **39**(11): pp. 1526–32.

[33] Tempest, H., et al., *Acupuncture in urological practice--a survey of urologists in England*. Complement Ther Med, 2011. **19**(1): pp. 27–31.

[34] Liu, B., et al., *Effect of blinding with a new pragmatic placebo needle: a randomized controlled crossover study*. Medicine (Baltimore), 2014. **93**(27): p. e200.

[35] Xu, H., et al., *A phase 1 clinical study on the efficacy of electroacupuncture for female patients with mild to moderate stress incontinence*. Chin J Trad Chin Med Phar, 2014. **29**(12): pp. 3755–8.

[36] Liu, Z., et al., *The efficacy and safety of electroacupuncture for women with pure stress urinary incontinence: study protocol for a multicenter randomized controlled trial*. Trials, 2013. **14**: p. 315.

[37] Su, T., et al., *The efficacy of electroacupuncture for the treatment of simple female stress urinary incontinence—comparison with pelvic floor muscle training: study protocol for a multicenter randomized controlled trial*. Trials, 2015. **16**: p. 45.

[38] Kaplan, S.A., et al., *Efficacy and safety of fesoterodine 8 mg in subjects with overactive bladder after a suboptimal response to tolterodine ER*. Int J Clin Pract, 2014. **68**(9): pp. 1065–73.

[39] Zhang, J., W. Cheng, and M. Cai, *Effects of electroacupuncture on overactive bladder refractory to anticholinergics: a single-blind randomised controlled trial*. Acupunct Med, 2015. 33(5):pp.368-74.

[40] Feng, Q., et al., *Quantity-effect relationship of electroacupuncture for urge incontinence: a multicenter randomized controlled trial*. J Acupunct Tuina Sci., 2012. **10**(1): pp. 49–53.

[41] Jin, C., X. Zhou, and R. Pang, *Effect of electro-acupuncture on mixed urinary incontinence*. J Clin Acupunct Med, 2013. **29**(6): pp. 59–60.

[42] Jin, C., X. Zhou, and R. Pang, *Effect of electroacupuncture combined with tolterodine on treating female mixed urinary incontinence*. J Wound Ostomy Continence Nurs, 2014. **41**(3): pp. 268–72.

[43] Gao, Y., et al., *Electroacupuncture for bladder function recovery in patients undergoing spinal anesthesia*. Evid Based Complement Alternat Med, 2014. **2014**: pp. 892619.

Chapter 4

Physiotherapy in Women with Urinary Incontinence

Özlem Çinar Özdemir and Mahmut Surmeli

Additional information is available at the end of the chapter

http://dx.doi.org/10.5772/64611

Abstract

Urinary incontinence is a complex and serious condition that can affect all age groups around the world. It is not only a serious medical condition but also an undeniable psychosocial problem creating embarrassment and negative self-perception, and it has a severe impact on a patient's quality of life. Today, there are wide different treatment options in urinary incontinence from surgery to conservative modalities. Among these, conservative management approaches are recommended as the first-line treatment to manage with urinary incontinence. The choice of the most suitable option to treat for urinary incontinence differs according to the underlying pathophysiological mechanism defining subtypes of urinary incontinence and severity of symptoms. In this chapter, we addressed the different components of physiotherapy management of urinary incontinence, including pelvic floor muscle training, electrical stimulation, biofeedback, vaginal cones, mechanical devices and magnetic stimulation. We concluded that the optimal physiotherapy care should be individualised to ensure applicability the clinic setting for each patient.

Keywords: urinary incontinence, pelvic floor muscle training, physiotherapy, biofeedback, women

1. Introduction

Urinary incontinence (UI) is defined by the International Continence Society as any involuntary leakage of urine [1]. It is one of the most common health problems seen in women of nearly all ages [2] and affects up to two-thirds of all women [3]. It is more frequent in women, and it is particularly common among those in residential care [4].

Female urinary incontinence is a complex situation [5]. It has been stated that UI might be indicative of a symptom, sign or condition. The symptom may indicate a state of loss of urinary control; the sign is the objective demonstration of urine leak, and the condition is the urodynamic demonstration and characterisation of urine loss [6].

UI should not be classified only as a serious medical condition leading to lower urinary tract infections and perineal rash but also as an undeniable psychosocial problem (**Figure 1**), creating embarrassment and negative self-perception [7]. This in turn affects a wide aspect of daily life, including the social, psychological, occupational, domestic, physical and sexual activities of women [2]. UI has been found to result in reduced social interactions and physical activities [8] and is commonly associated with poor self-rated health [9], impaired psychological well-being, sexual relationships, decreased quality of life (QoL) [10] and increased depressive symptoms [11]. It may restrict employment and educational or leisure opportunities leading to embarrassment and exclusion [12].

There is a wide range of literature on the prevalences of UI [13, 14]. This can be explained by the differences in the definition of UI, in epidemiologic methodology, and in the demographic characteristics among the studies [13–15]. About 25% of young women, 44–57% of middle-aged and postmenopausal women, and about 75% of older women experience some involuntary urine loss [16]. In the 5th International Consultation on Incontinence (2012), it is stated that the prevalence of UI in the population varies between 30% and 60% in middle-aged and older women and it increases with age. In addition, the prevalence of daily UI changes from 5 to 15%, and it rises over 15% in women aged above 70 years [14]. Although these ranges of prevalence of UI are usually underestimated in the clinical setting, since patients often fail to bring the condition to the attention of their physicians. It is estimated that only one in four symptomatic women seeks help for this problem [17].

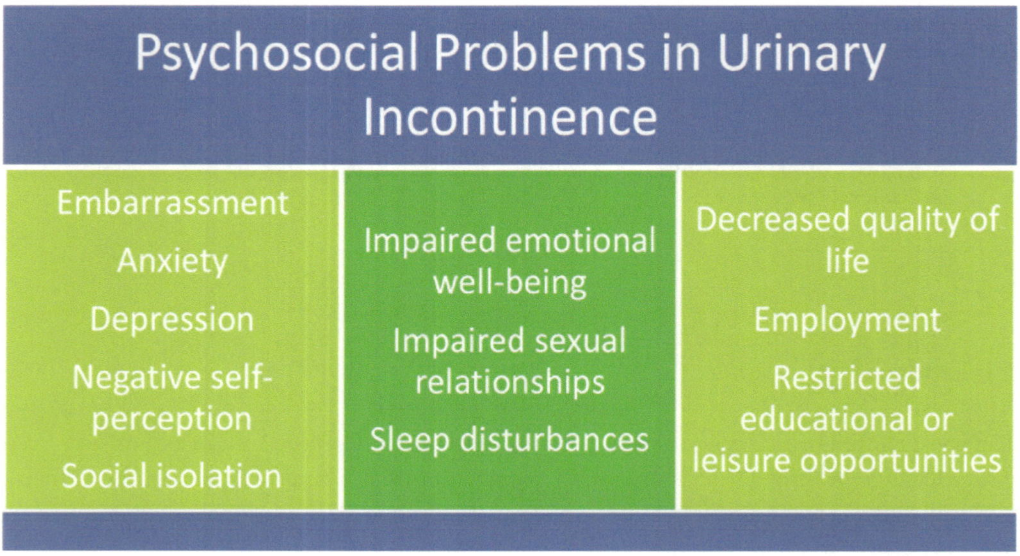

Figure 1. Psycho-social problems seen in urinary incontinence.

http://dx.doi.org/10.5772/64611

UI affects not only the sufferers but also their family, friends and the general public, due to its associated medical costs and social stigma [18]. UI is generally not related directly to survival but affects the QoL of the patients, causes mental distress and reduces day-to-day activities. When the treatment for UI results in the alleviation or cure of the condition, the distress can be eliminated and return to a normal life is possible [19]. In general, the choice of treatment primarily depends on the balance between efficacy and the associated complications. A variety of effective conservative treatment modalities are available to manage symptoms of UI [20].

There are several risk factors associated with UI in women (**Figure 2**). These include age, obesity, race/ethnicity, childbirth, oral hormonal therapy, prior hysterectomy, cognitive impairment, mobility impairment, diabetes [21], history of pelvic and perineal surgery [5] pregnancy, pelvic floor trauma after vaginal delivery and menopause [22]. UI may also occur as a result of a number of abnormalities of function of the lower urinary tract, or as a result of other illnesses [23], use of diuretics, sedentary lifestyles, caffeinated and carbonated drinks, severe and/or chronic cough resulting from, for example, chronic bronchitis or smoking, bladder stones, short urethra and hypoestrogenemia. These conditions may lead to urinary leakage under different situations [24].

The different types of incontinences are distinguished by their baseline mechanisms [16]. There are three major subtypes of UI: stress urinary incontinence (SUI), urge urinary incontinence (UUI) (urgent need to void) and mixed urinary incontinence (MUI) [25]. SUI is characterised by involuntary loss of urine without any previous feeling of a need to void, which occurs while under a physical stress like cough, lifting something heavy or any other physical activities [5]. UUI is characterised by an involuntary leakage accompanied by or immediately preceded by urgency that is difficult to defer followed by an irresistible need to void [25], resulting in uncontrollable leakage of urine [5]. MUI refers to the involuntary leakage associated with variable proportions of urgency and also with exertion, effort, sneezing or coughing

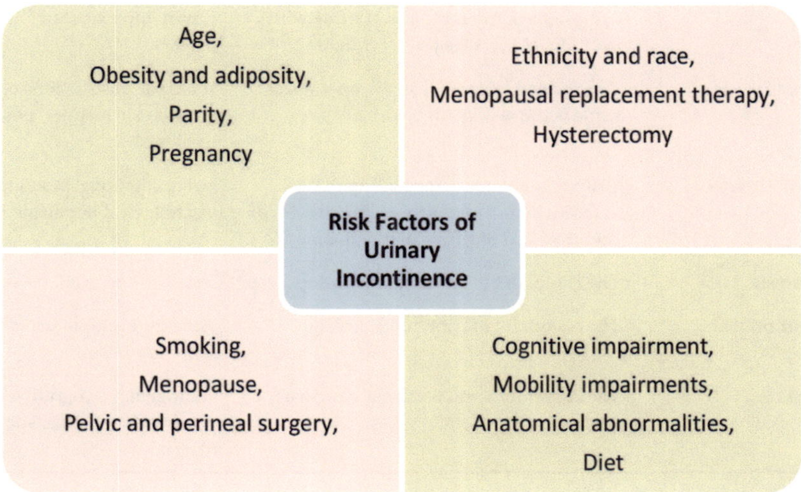

Figure 2. Risk factors for urinary incontinence.

[25–27]. These definitions reflect the consensus definitions developed by the International Urogynecological Association and International Continence Society [27]. There are also less common categories of UI. These include total incontinence which is associated with urinary tract fistula or ectopic ureter, functional incontinence, which is associated with psychiatric or mobility disorders, overflow incontinence, post-micturition dribble, radiotherapy and climacturia [28], nocturnal enuresis, continuous UI and UI due to idiopathic or neurogenic detrussor [29]. Different types of incontinence, their definitions and possible causes are given in **Table 1** [14, 30].

There exists a wide range of treatment options to treat UI from surgical interventions to conservative modalities. Current guidelines recommend conservative management that is defined as interventions that do not involve treatment with drugs or surgery targeted to the type of incontinence [23, 31], as the first-line therapy in UI [13, 31, 32]. Therefore, there is an option for conservative management, and physiotherapy, particularly for women who have not completed their childbearing and for those with mild symptoms [33]. Physical therapy modalities have been in use for several decades to treat UI and other lower urinary tract symptoms. They have been adopted by several disciplines and are implemented in many different ways [34].

Types of urinary incontinence		
Types	**Definitions**	**Pathophysiology and causes**
Stress urinary incontinence	Loss of urine during physical movements (coughing, sneezing, jumping, lifting, exercising)	Weakness of pelvic floor muscles or urethral sphincters, post-urologic surgery
Urge urinary incontinence	Leakage of urine at unexpected times accompanied by, or immediately preceded by a strong desire to void	Detrusor overactivity (uninhibited bladder contractions), neurologic disorders
Mixed urinary incontinence	Involuntary leakage associated with symptoms of urgency; loss of urine with exertion, effort, sneezing or coughing	Mixed etiology of stress and urge urinary incontinence
Overflow incontinence	Unexpected leakage of small amounts of urine because of a full bladder	Anatomic obstructions of urethra, a contractile bladder, neurogenic problems
Functional incontinence	Urinary accidents associated with the inability to toilet because of impairment of cognitive and or physical functioning	Severe cognitive, mobility or psychological impairments
Nocturnal enuresis	The complaint of loss of urine during sleep	Genetics, nocturnal polyuria, idiopatic
Continuous incontinence	The complaint of continuous leakage	Diabetes, multiple sclerosis, blockage of urinary tracts
Total incontinence	The continuous and total loss of urinary control	Neurogenic or cognitive problems, vesicovaginal fistula, spinal cord injuries

Table 1. Types of urinary incontinence, their definitions and pathophysiologic mechanisms with possible causes.

The main purpose of the conservative management is to strengthen the pelvic floor and modulate behaviours that influence bladder function, whereas pharmacological therapies targets innervating the bladder and sphincter [16, 22]. The aim of conservative rehabilitation therapy is to stabilise the urethra by increasing pelvic floor muscle (PFM) strength (force-generating capacity). Pelvic floor muscles (PFM) strength is important to support and stabilize bladder neck and urethra [15].

The researchers and patients see improvements in UI in different ways. Sufferers define improvement according to reduced lifestyle limitations or healing overall perception of bladder symptoms, especially recovery of urine leakage. In the view of the researchers, an improvement is a decrease in the amount of urine lost during pad tests, or any statistically significant decrease in the frequency of UI episodes [35].

There are some conservative therapy modalities to obtain improvement in patients with UI. Among these techniques, pelvic floor muscle training (PFMT), electrical stimulation (ES), biofeedback, magnetic stimulation (MS) and vaginal cones (VCs) are mostly used as a therapy method before surgical options in some situations. Training and strengthening the PFMs is recommended as the first-line management for women with SUI, UUI and MUI [15, 23].

2. Pelvic floor muscle training

Pelvic floor muscle exercises (PFME) offers a possible reprieve from UI [36]. Therefore, PFMT remains a key factor in the prevention and treatment of UI [14]. This conservative therapy appears to have no significant side effects and help in improving symptoms. It can therefore be considered as the first choice of treatment for UI in women. The guideline states that pelvic floor exercises have been found to be effective in the treatment of incontinence in more than 50% female patients [23, 37]. It is commonly recommended for the treatment of patients with SUI or MUI [38]. Less commonly, it can be used for UUI [39]. It has been demonstrated that PFME can improve the strength of the female PFMs contraction, increase intraurethral pressure and elevate the urethra to maintain continence [40, 41]. Through the agency of all these benefits, symptoms of SUI in women result in improvement. In addition, fast-repeated contractions of the levator ani musculature have been demonstrated to stimulate the sacral reflex arch to suppress urinary urgency and frequency and improve UUI symptoms [41, 42].

PFMT for the management of UI has been described in several ancient texts of China, India, Greece and Rome [37, 43]. It was thought that strengthening this group of muscles would promote health, longevity, spiritual development and sexual health. The first report of PFMT in modern medicine dates back to 1936, when a paper by Margaret Morris described tensing and relaxing of the PFMs as a preventative and treatment option for urinary and faecal incontinence [37]. Subsequently, PFMT was introduced to the British physiotherapy profession. However, PFMT was popularised by Arnold Kegel for the management of UI in 1948 and has since remained as a first-line conservative measure [44–46]. In his paper "Progressive resistance exercise in the functional restoration of the perineal muscles", he reported the successful treatment in patients with SUI [47], and the term Kegel exercise, as a common misnomer for pelvic floor exercises, came into existence [37]. As mentioned above, PFMT commonly recommended and used for the treatment for SUI or MUI especially with SUI symptoms [44, 48, 49] and pelvic organ prolapse (POP) [50], as the first choice of treatment for SUI/MUI [38]. Less commonly, it is used for the treatment of UUI [32, 39, 48, 49].

PFMT is mostly aimed to improve the function of the PFM in terms of strength which is the maximum force generated by a muscle in a single contraction, endurance which is the ability to perform repetitive contractions or to sustain a single contraction over time and coordination that is muscular activity prior to effort and on exertion, or any combinations of these, thus providing thereby maximum support to the pelvic organs, especially the bladder neck and the proximal urethra, before and during an increase in intra-abdominal pressure, to prevent urine leakage [39]. PFM strength training results in an improved support to the bladder neck and proximal urethra, which have been observed to be poorly supported in some patients with UI. This is achieved by elevating the position of the levator ani muscle through muscle hypertrophy and increased muscle stiffness [39, 51].

There are 12 striated muscles arranged in three layers in the pelvic floor. These three layers consist of the endopelvic fascia, the levator ani muscles and the perineal membrane, respectively. The endopelvic fascia is the connective tissue floor of the pelvis, extending between the viscera to the pelvic walls. It is considered as first layer of pelvic floor. The levator ani muscles and their fascia are considered as second layer which is also referring as the pelvic diagram. It serves as horizontal sheet with anterior hiatus in the midline. The urethra, the vagina and the rectum pass through within this hiatus. If this layer is disrupted during parturition, there will have a consequent effect on all the three structures. The last layer is the perineal membrane (or in other words urogenital diaphragm) and lies at the hymeneal ring. In females it does not complete due to the position of the vagina. Thus, this membrane provides some weak support for the urethra. Lying under the perineal membrane are the ischiocavernosus, bulbocavernosus and superficial transverse perineal muscles [52].

The PFMs consist of muscle fibres, of which 70% are slow-twitch type 1, that is, fatigue-resistant fibres maintaining static tone and 30% are fast-twitch type 2 that is fatigue-prone fibres being capable of active contraction. In some situations like aging, inactivity and nerve innervation damage, there might be a decrease in the proportion of the fast-twitch fibres [53]. Doing exercise can increase PFM strength, durability and responsiveness [47, 54].

In order to prevent UI, PFMT works in several ways. In females, the bladder neck and urethra are supported by the PFMs. Just before intra-abdominal pressure begins to increase, PFMs is activated and this activation is maintained during increased intra-abdominal pressure. Contraction of PFMs pressures the urethra to the pubic symphysis. Consequently, the urethral resistance increases and this increased resistance prevents involuntary loss of urine. It is demonstrated that urethral and bladder neck descent and leakage of urine can be prevented by a well-timed contraction when intra-abdominal pressure increases. The repetitive exercises which are done regularly cause muscle hypertrophy, improve the urethral resistance and help to prevent POP [50].

PFMs integrity appears to play an important role in the continence mechanism. Therefore, there is a biological rationale in improving the use of PFMT in preventing and treating UI in women [47]. There are two main biological reasons for using PFMT. Firstly, a voluntary contraction before and during a cough has been shown to effectively reduce urinary leakage during cough (a manoeuvre termed "The Knack") [55]. Secondly, increase in PFMs strength is thought to beef up long-lasting structural support to the pelvis by ascending the levator plate. This is also enhanced by hypertrophy of the muscles which increases further the stiffness of the PFMs and connective tissues [51]. Thus, perineal descent during increased intra-abdominal pressure could be prevented by improving the PFM strength. Improvement in the PFM strength may also facilitate PFMs before and during the effort, thereby reducing SUI in women. Given the above biological rationale, while treating SUI, the focus of any PFMT should be improving the timing of the contraction, strength and stiffness of the PFMs [48].

PFME, which includes repetitively selective voluntary contraction and relaxation of the specific PFMs [27], is used to increase the strength of the PFMs and periurethral muscles. This in turn improves the efficiency of the supportive function by immobilising the urethra and improves the sphincteric function by increasing the intraurethral closure pressure during physical activities [51, 56]. The movement is a voluntary inward and upward contraction and squeeze of the pelvic floor. The basic principles of muscle training according to the American College of Sports Medicine are based on progressive overload, specificity and periodisation, which need to be incorporated into any resistance training programme in order to achieve maximum results [48]. As the pelvic floor is entirely composed of striated muscles, the principles of strength training for the striated muscle can also be applied to PFMs [37, 48]. During the PFMT, the purpose of progressive overload is to gradually increase the intensity of the exercises and the number of repetitions throughout the exercise programme. By submaximal loads, the speed of the repetitions should be adjusted according to the desired goal. For endurance improvement and power training or lengthened for strength, the rest periods should be shortened. In the end, the overall volume of training should be increased gradually [37].

Different studies have recommended different number of contractions ranging from 8 to 12 contractions three times a day to 20 contractions four times a day and up to as many as 200 contractions per day [37]. To obtain increased muscle strength of PFMs, it is necessary to apply a method, named as the progression model. This method requires doing repetition from 8 to 12 times with maximum contractions at moderate velocity and 1 or 2 min breaks between sets. Moreover, number of initial trainings which were two to three times in a week should be increased to four to five times per week. Additionally, as a person can achieve the current workload for one to two repetitions over the determined number, the initial work load should be increased about 2–10%. In order to increase muscle endurance, the progression model suggests the need for light to moderate loads (40–60% of maximal load) with high repetitions (>15) and short rest periods (<90 s) for endurance training. In PFMT, progression can be achieved by changing positions from gravity-free to antigravity or through the introduction of cones into the exercise sessions. Finally, if it is desired to obtain better outcomes according to progression model, velocity and coordination training ("The Knack") should include the use of repetitive, voluntary PFMs contractions in response to specific situations; for example, prior to and during coughing, lifting an object or jumping [48]. The National

Institute for Health and Care Excellence (NICE) recommends PFMT comprising at least eight contractions three times daily for at least 3 months as the first-line therapy for the women with SUI [23]. The American College of Obstetricians and Gynaecologists also recommends PFMT as the first-line therapy for the women with SUI and states that PFMT is more effective than ES or VCs [57].

There are different recommended postures that are adopted during the prescribed exercise regimen. These postures include sitting, kneeling, standing, lying down and standing with legs astride. There are huge variations in the recommended duration of the prescribed regimen starting from 1 week to 6 months, with 3 months being most frequently recommended. Across studies the number of contractions ranges from 8 to 12 contractions three times a day, to 20 contractions four times a day, to as many as 200 contractions per day [37]. NICE recommends a trial of supervised pelvic floor exercises, consisting of at least eight contractions three times a day for a minimum of 3 months, as the first-line treatment for UI [37, 58]. The recommended supervised PFMT by The International Consultation on Incontinence Committee for women with SUI is 8–12 weeks before reassessment with a possible referral for further management, if the patient does not improved desirably [37, 59]. The intensity of the contraction seems to be more important than frequency of training [60].

To obtain better outcomes from PFMT, PFMs may be activated together with the abdominal muscle. It is known that active contraction of the transversus abdominis (TA) muscle is associated with co-activation of the PFMs. However, PFMs are not raised in all women by the TA muscle contraction. In recent studies, it is suggested that the relationship between PFM and TA muscle vary between continent and incontinent women. In incontinent women with SUI, TA muscle contraction with the PFM being displaced less during the contraction of TA muscle as compared to the continent women [37].

Among the conservative treatment options, this conservative therapy appears to have no side effects and enables improvement in symptoms; it can therefore be considered as a first choice of treatment for UI in women [37].

3. Electrical stimulation

Another popular intervention used by physiotherapists to reduce UI is ES. It is one of the first-line conservative treatment option for female UI and widely used in the management of it. ES physiologically produces muscle hypertrophy, normalises the reflex activity of the lower urinary tract and increases circulation to muscles and the capillary system [7, 61]. It may also increase conscious awareness of the action of PFMs to provide an improved ability to perform a voluntary muscle contraction. With regard to a recent systematic review, ES does not differ from sham stimulation or PFME in terms of improvement in UI [62]. However, ES is a priority for women with difficulty in contracting the PFMs initially [7, 61].

ES is a therapeutic option for patients with UI and based on the application of electrical impulses to the peripheral nerves [63]. In 1963, ES of the muscles of the pelvic floor was first offered by Caldwell to address urinary and faecal incontinence. Since then, clinical trials

http://dx.doi.org/10.5772/64611

showed some efficacy in treating UI particularly in SUI, UUI and MUI [31, 64]. It includes the application of ES to the suprapubical, transvaginal, sacral and tibial nerves [64] and denoted as functional ES [31]. The process of sacral nerve stimulation includes implantation of a wire electrode in one of the sacral foramina, usually S3, which is then connected to a stimulator device. In most cases, it is useful for refractory UI and idiopathic urinary retention [65, 66]. ES of the tibial nerve is a peripheral non-implantable method, which can be applied percutaneously with a needle or transcutaneously with a stick-on electrocardiograph-type electrode [31, 65]. In this, S2-S4 crossroads of the sacral nerve plexus delivers neuromodulation to pelvic floor through the less invasive route of the posterior tibial nerve. There are projections in this area to the sacral nerve plexus. A feedback loop is generated, modulating bladder innervations [31, 67]. The main of suprapubical ES is to make a direct stimulation of S3 nerve roots, in order to inhibit the detrusor activity, equivalently to the sacral ES, but is less invasive [31, 68].

ES is generally directed with a removable device through vaginal or anal stimulation [69]. The electrodes can be implantable or non-implantable, and the ES can be of long or short duration [31]. The electrodes are placed in the vaginal or rectal canals in such a way as to acquire direct contact with a remarkable amount of afferent nerve fibres of the pudendal nerve [70]. It is necessary to partially or totally innervate the pudendal nerve so that nerve stimulation can occur [70, 71]. The advantage of this therapy is that it does not ask for voluntary patient effort; however, the passive muscle contractions are generally weaker than the voluntary ones [63].

The mechanism of action of this modality relies on the ES to induce hypertrophy of skeletal PFM [25, 72], which cannot be achieved by voluntary muscle contractions via reflex contractions, while activating the detrusor inhibitory reflex arc [25, 72]. The important outcomes of electrical stimulation are the reorganisation of spinal reflex and regulation of cortical activity, which are related to the mechanism of action of this therapy [73]. The mechanism of action of ES is to promote bladder relaxation by inhibiting the parasympathetic motor neurons. Other studies reported that transvaginal ES causes contractions of the pelvic floor, increasing the number of muscle fibres with rapid contraction, which are responsible for continence in conditions of stress [31, 65].

The aim of ES in the treatment of patients with SUI appears to improve the function of the PFMs [74] by stimulating its contraction, with the goal of achieving a training effect to ensure that the pelvic floor will provide adequate support with the advancement in PFM strength to prevent urine loss during an increase in intra-abdominal pressure [75]. While for women with UUI, the intention seems to be to inhibit detrusor overactivity [74].

The principle of ES for the treatment of SUI based on the delivery of electrical impulses to directly trigger reflex contraction of the PFMs through the pudendal nerve and by activating three concomitant central actions. These concomitant actions are activation of hypogastric inhibitory fibres to the bladder, central inhibition of pelvic outflow to the bladder and central inhibition of the ascending afferent pathway from the bladder. Voluntary pelvic floor muscle contraction does not lead to the activation of this reflex pathway [72, 76].

ES can evoke direct contractions of the PFM in patients with detrusor overactivity or symptoms of urgency and UUI. The contractions stimulate afferent fibres of the pudendal nerve going to the sacral spinal cord [2], and this stimulation induces a reflex contraction of the striated paraurethral and periurethral muscles, accompanied by a simultaneous reflex inhibition of the detrusor muscle [69, 72, 76, 77]. This response leads to a reflexive decrease in the feeling or sensation of urgency and inhibits parasympathetic activity at the level of the sacral micturition centre in the sacral cord that eventually reduces involuntary detrusor contractions and reflexively activates the striated periurethral musculature [2]. Peripheral innervation of the PFMs must at least be partly intact to gain a therapeutic effect of pelvic floor stimulation in women with detrusor overactivity [78].

There are major inconsistencies that exist between several electrostimulation protocols, partly due to a lack of understanding of the physiological principles of electrostimulation and the way it could contribute to recuperation from SUI in women. Different forms of electrostimulation are distinguished in physical therapy, brief maximal stimulation, which is usually performed at a physical therapy centre and prolonged, low-intensity electrostimulation, which can also be performed at home. The potential side effects of electrostimulation include pain and tissue damage; electrostimulation is contra-indicated if patient is using a pacemaker or in case of pregnancy [61]. Stimulation parameters have been defined on the basis of neurophysiological and clinical studies (**Figure 3**) [72, 79].

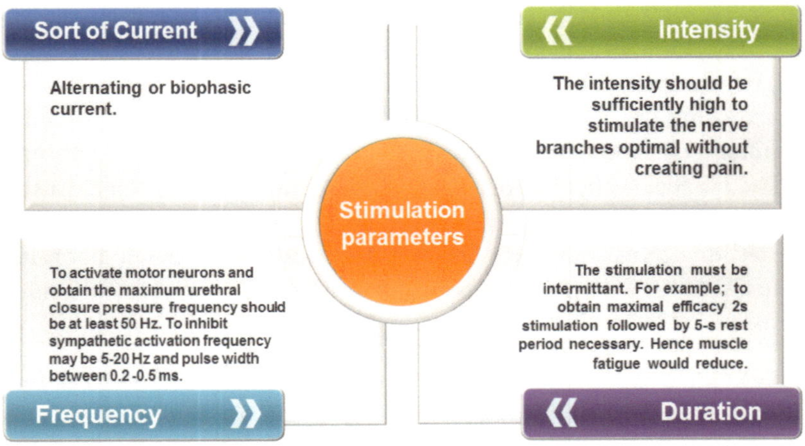

Figure 3. Stimulation parameters of electrical stimulation.

3.1. PFME and electrical stimulation

Patients with very weak PFMs often have difficulty identifying and activating their muscles to improve symptoms of SUI. In this situation, ES can be useful to activate PFMs. To improve the efficacy of PFMT, it is combined with ES. Hence, combination of these might facilitate training by helping patients to better identify and strengthen their muscles, leading to better treatment outcomes [34]. The sense of contracting the PFMs is a useful reminder to the patient of the sensation that should be perceived, and they are encouraged to actively try to contract the PFM during ES [33, 79].

It may be that electrical stimulation is particularly appropriate for patients who are initially unable to contract their PFM, but once active contraction is achieved, PFME may be more effective [80, 81].

In most physiotherapy practices, electrical stimulation is used for partially paralysed muscles and to stimulate the activity when the patients are unable to contract it voluntarily. Most physiotherapists prefer stop using ES and continue with regular muscle training when the patient can contract voluntarily [82].

In general, there are two main mechanisms by which ES is believed to work. One of these ES in the form of neurostimulation aims to stimulate motor efferent fibres of the pudendal nerve, which elicits a direct response from the effector organ, for instance, a contraction of the PFMs [70, 83, 84]. Other mechanism of these, ES in the form of neuromodulation aims to remodel reflex loops, for instance, the detrusor inhibition reflex by stimulating afferent nerve fibres of the pudendal nerve that influence these reflex loops via the spinal cord [70, 85].

4. Biofeedback

One of the recent definitions of biofeedback is giving an indication on bodily processes using an external sensor within a group of experimental procedures, mostly in order to readjust the measured quality [82]. Another definition is coexisting, simultaneous or terminal biological feedback of biological signals allowing a person to determine and modify a bodily function of which they are usually unacquainted [86, 87].

Assisting patients for the determination and also their exercise the PFM properly is accepted as the main objective of biofeedback [34]. Although it is not a therapy in itself, it is possible to be applied in the treatment of patients with SUI for several reasons. Firstly, it provides them an indication of their PFM activity at rest, in contraction and relaxation modes; secondly, it gives not only the strength of individual contractions of the PFMs but also the strength of the contracting PFMs or the way in which certain muscles contract and the direction of contraction. Since biofeedback gives information related with the learning and controlling the functions of the activity of striated muscles through varied audio-visual techniques, it can also be used to educate a certain patient suffering SUI, about the selective contraction of their PFMs. Introducing a sensor or electrode into the vagina or rectum is the most common method to provide biofeedback. By this way, the vaginal or rectal pressure or the electromyogram (EMG) signal of the sphincter muscle is recorded. The visual or acoustic information about the pressures measured and/or the EMG signals are sent to the patients, thus enabling them to see the magnitude of the force being generated by the PFMs and to know if this force has reached its maximum level. The technique can also be used to visualise progress, which obviously motivates patients to keep exercising (biofeedback device is shown in **Figure 4**). Biofeedback is not a therapy to be applied solely; however, it is possible that a combination of biofeedback and PFMT is beneficial for decreasing the reluctant leakage of urine in SUI suffering patients. The efficacy and professional knowledge of a physical therapist plays a significant role on the effective results of biofeedback usage [61].

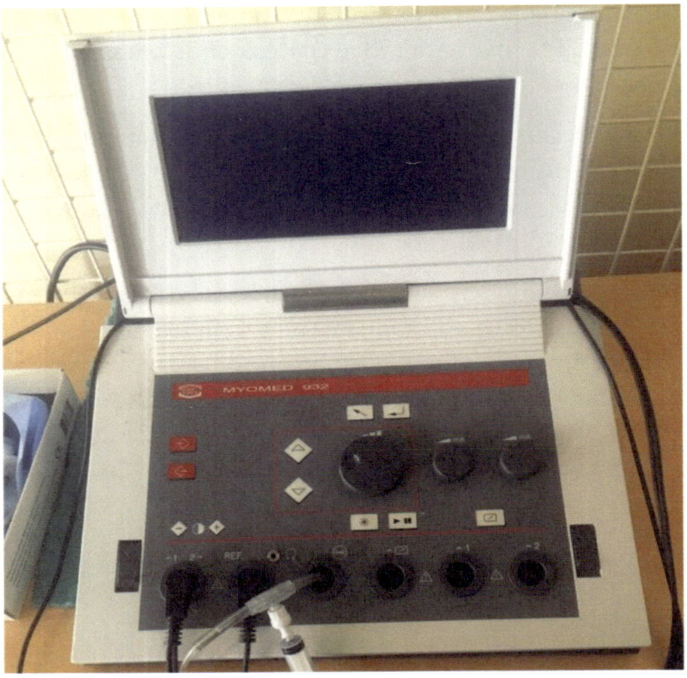

Figure 4. Biofeedback device.

Even though biofeedback technology is accepted as a proven technique assuring proper muscle control, it needs specific equipment as well as professional expertise, which results in longer time period and higher financial cost [34]. The contribution of the field of psychology has been required for the development of the biofeedback equipment; hence, varied forms of stress are needed to be measured through sweating, heart rate and blood pressure. Using vaginal palpation and clinical observation during the instruction of accurate contraction was indispensable for Kegel's training protocol [47]. During Kegel's exercise, as biofeedback, a combination of PFMT and vaginal squeeze pressure measurement was used. Nowadays, in clinical practice, wide ranges of biofeedback apparatus are in use [82]. Biofeedback devices vary considerably. They can be inserted into the rectum or vagina or placed on the perineum. Many of the biofeedback devices addressed in this review are either air- or water-filled balloons inserted into the rectum or vagina to measure pressure. Vaginal, anal and intra-abdominal pressure can be measured regulated by the balloon catheters' quantity and induction. The other main group of biofeedback devices measures electrical activity (i.e. electromyography) via surface metal electrodes on vaginal or anal probes. Displaying movement, such as moving bladder neck upwards, is another claim of biofeedback, which can be provided by ultrasound real time images [87].

A number of studies have tried to figure out which method is more beneficial to teach pelvic floor muscle control: biofeedback training or digital palpation with verbal feedback. However, they are not consistent, and there is need to studies coming up with a clear benefit biofeedback to a PFMT program [34, 87]. Biofeedback could be implemented for patients who cannot identify their muscles well by other methods. Additionally, it is suggested that behavioural methods can be used more widely particularly in settings where biofeedback is not accessible [34].

Biofeedback-assisted exercises present the advantage of additional acoustic and visual guidance for the patient, which makes it easier for them to learn and perform the exercises appropriately [88, 89]. Another advantage of biofeedback is to help the women who have difficulty in isolating their PFM during training. Furthermore, patients who can identify the PFM often find that the required daily exercise routine is burdensome. Most of the patients fail to comply with the PFMT for a long-term [89, 90]. ES is a non-invasive, passive treatment that produces a muscle contraction [89, 91]. PFM contraction by indirect nerve stimulation and polysynaptic reflex responses is caused by transvaginal electrical stimulation (TES) [89, 90, 92]. As long as performed accurately, PFMT results more effective than ES because of the indirect stimulation and reflexive contraction. Biofeedback-assisted PFMT and TES have been used together to improve therapeutic effect [89].

4.1. PFME along with biofeedback

In the field of urology or urogynaecological, the term "biofeedback" is often used to classify a method different from PFMT. Biofeedback is helpful for training and evaluating response from a single PFMs activity. In the area of PFMT, with both vaginal and anal surface EMG, urethral and vaginal squeeze pressure measurements have been utilised with the purpose of making the patients to know better their muscle functions and to enhance and motivate patients' effort through training [82, 93]. PFME are possible to be supported by biofeedback, since it gives relative information on unconscious physiological processes. Provided information establishes the primary support for active self-control processes under observation [69].

In SUI treatment, biofeedback could be used in combination with PFMT to demonstrate PFM activity at rest, on activity and in relaxation period. In addition, it represents the ability of a person (by electromyogram) or overall (pressure measurement) PFM contraction. However, combination of PFME with biofeedback is not more effective than PFMT which is done solo [75, 94, 95]. Although each treatment modalities are useful by itself, it is probable that biofeedback added value in SUI patients suffering unawareness and/or control of the pelvic floor, quick improvement from the beginning phase and motivate the patients for the exercise [60, 75].

The exact contraction may be verified by using biofeedback or manual palpation. In women, biofeedback is applied by using small electrodes which are placed around the anus or by using an internal vaginal electrode. Biofeedback allows women to see their muscle output during an exercise instantly. However, information available in the literature suggests that PFME with biofeedback is not as effective as PFME applied alone. On the other hand, combining PFME with biofeedback can be clinically beneficial and acceptable treatment procedure for certain groups of woman. A practical strategy may be to begin with PFME with biofeedback for those who might have difficulty in understanding how to contract or are unable to contract the PFM. Biofeedback can also be used to teach the correct form of PFME [7].

5. Vaginal cones

PFMT is the main approach of conservative (non-surgical) treatment in SUI. It is based on strength training or identification or both for the PFM to overcome weakness by increasing the support of urethra and bladder, and improving sphincteric action of muscles around the urethra [96].

On the other hand, this muscles group seems rather difficult to be determined and controlled by women. Moreover, these muscles are below par to the training completion; hence, it will probably require other intervention modalities [25]. In addition, incorrect PFMs contractions can make the incontinence worse [97]. While considering these reasons, weighted VCs were developed as a method of strengthening and testing the function of the PFM [98].

Plevnik introduced the usage of VCs in 1985 [98]. His aim was to strengthen PFMs with the VCs by inserting them in the vagina higher to the pelvic floor musculature [63]. Theoretically, when a cone is placed in the vagina, the PFMs need to be contracted to prevent the cone slipping out [96]. The sensation of losing the cones from the vagina provides a strong sensory feedback and prompts a PFM contraction in order to retain the cone [74]. In order to keep the cone inside the vagina, these muscles are needed to be contracted. Same sized but different weighted set of VCs are given to the patient and she is asked to insert a cone of increasingly heavier weight until she can hold the earlier lighter one [61, 63]. Developing muscular overload is provided by the cones. During the exercise process, the patient inserts the selected cone intravaginally, above the level of the levatores muscle plate, using a standardised procedure, and tries to hold the cone in place for up to 15 min by contracting her PFMs [61, 99]. If a positive result is obtained twice in a row, the training can be continued with the subsequent heavier cone. A training based on this principle is believed to strengthen the PFMs under simultaneous proprioceptive feedback [61].

There are some perceived advantages of the cones over traditional methods of training the PFMs [96, 100–102] and these are demonstrated in **Table 2**.

The probability of maintaining sensory-motor biofeedback brings about the certain advantages of strengthening the PFMs by using VCs [103]. This sensory-motor biofeedback can possibly maximise the neural gains as the greatest activation and synchronisation of the motor units [104]. And hence, the vaginal cone usage would support an accelerated improvement in muscle strength through neural mechanisms, followed by muscle hypertrophy in response to resistance training with progression of the cone weight [104, 105].

Although working out with cones has been criticised as not being suitable for all women especially with a narrow and scarred vagina or individual admissibility and weight of the cone may not represent the strength of PFM, weighted VCs has been shown to increase the strength of the PFM and has been found to have similar efficacy in comparison with PFME and ES. However, it enjoys the benefit of requiring less time to train for its application with need of only one or two consultations, being able to be used without supervision, providing a form of biofeedback and helping muscle synchronisation with increases in abdominal pressure [96, 104]

http://dx.doi.org/10.5772/64611

1	**Advantages of the cones**
2	The exercise is individualised for each woman
3	Less time is needed to teach women to use the cones than to teach PFMT
4	It does not take much time to insert and remove cones
5	The use of VCs can be self-taught, and they can be used without supervision and vaginal examination
6	The graded increases in cone weight represent improvement in muscle strength and motivates women to continue
7	Usually only one consultation is needed
8	Cones can be used in self-instruction of conventional PFMT
	The cones provide a form of biofeedback as the sensation of one slipping out induces a PFM contraction which may both strengthen muscles and help to synchronize muscle contraction with increases in abdominal pressure

Table 2. Advantages of the weighted vaginal cones.

6. Mechanical devices

Vaginal support prostheses have been in use for a long time. Although these devices are primarily used for POP, there has been some interest in developing those specific for SUI. Some potential advantages of these vaginal support devices include their potential to be applicable to the majority of the incontinent patients, mild side effects and non-requirement of any specific testing (e.g. urodynamic testing). Conversely, these devices do not definitively treat the problem, and if the problem worsens, the patient health may require a surgical intervention. Furthermore, these devices have no correction effect on intrinsic sphincter deficiency in reality, and may not help patients with hypermobility. There is a recent Cochrane review looked at seven trials involving over 700 women [106]. Three are small trials comparing mechanical devices (intravaginal such as pessary, sponge or tampon-like device) with no treatment suggested that use of a mechanical device might be better than no treatment; however, results were not conclusive. Urethral plugs passively occlude and/or coapt the urethra, but require removal for voiding. Overall results of the studies of Staskin and associates were generally favourable [107]. Although urethral inserts can work for most of the women with pure SUI, the shortcoming that these devices must be removed and reinserted with each void is not accepted by most of them [25].

7. Magnetic stimulation

Magnetic stimulation is a novel approach, coming up in recent years. The United States Food and Drug Administration approved MS as a conservative treatment for UI in 1998 [29, 108]. Ever since, to evaluate its efficacy in UI, more than 50 clinical experiments have been conducted worldwide [29, 109]. However, the multitude of information was overwhelming. According to clinicians, there is a need to compile these informations so that evidence-based decisions could be taken [29].

To use of MS there must be special chair. An electric current is passed around a metal coil, generating an electromagnetic field. When the person exposed to this field, electric current is generated in tissues. Thus, PFMs is stimulated by the MS in a similar way to ES. In this case, the patients are required neither to undress nor to insert electrodes, as the electromagnetic fields spread easily through tissues causing ES [110, 111]. It has an armed treatment chair for the patient to sit comfortably and a compact control unit (**Figure 5**). It contains a generator, control buttons, a monitoring screen and modem, and is equipped with automatic payment system for treatment sessions. The stimulation coil is situated underneath the treatment chair to ensure direct focus on PFMs [108, 111].

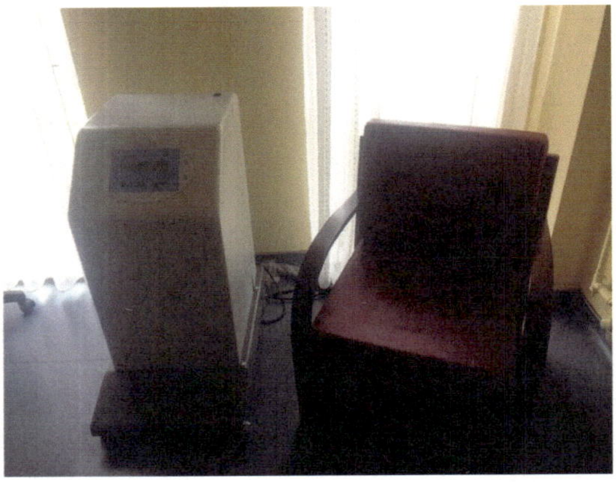

Figure 5. Equipment of magnetic stimulation.

It has not been established that the optimal frequency and pulse duration in MS yet. However, using more than 50 Hz has been reported as necessary to achieve an adequate PFMs contraction for treatment of SUI [109], and 38–40 Hz and less than 10–20 Hz for UUI [29, 112, 113].

Conservative therapy should be considered prior to the initiation of medical or surgical treatment of UI. Because of its demonstrated efficacy, low risk and apparent low cost, published clinical guidelines recommend that conservative management. Pelvic floor muscle training is recommended as first-line conservative management for treating urinary incontinence. Additional physical therapies, such as electrical stimulation, biofeedback or magnetic stimulation can be considered in women who cannot actively contract their pelvic floor muscles, in order to aid motivation and adherence to therapy. Physiotherapists need to understand the nature of the urinary incontinence, the influence prognostic factors and the principal of therapy modalities.

Author details

Özlem Çinar Özdemir* and Mahmut Surmeliv

*Address all correspondence to: ozlemcinar314@hotmail.com

School of Physical Therapy and Rehabilitation, Abant Izzet Baysal University, Bolu, Turkey

References

[1] Abrams P, Blaivas JG, Stanton SL, Andersen JT. Standardisation of terminology of lower urinary tract function. Neurourology and Urodynamics. 1988;7(5):403–27.

[2] Güler Ty, N. Urinary incontinence in women and physical theraphy. DPÜ Fen Bilimleri Enstitüsü Degisi. 2006.

[3] Smith PP, McCrery RJ, Appell RA. Current trends in the evaluation and management of female urinary incontinence. Canadian Medical Association Journal. 2006;175(10):1233–40.

[4] Hunskaar S, Arnold E, Burgio K, Diokno A, Herzog A, Mallett V. Epidemiology and natural history of urinary incontinence. International Urogynecology Journal. 2000;11(5):301–19.

[5] Legendre G, Ringa V, Fauconnier A, Fritel X. Menopause, hormone treatment and urinary incontinence at midlife. Maturitas. 2013;74(1):26–30.

[6] Bristow SE, Hilton P. Assessment and investigations for urinary incontinence. Best Practice & Research Clinical Obstetrics & Gynaecology. 2000;14(2):227–49.

[7] Ghaderi F, Oskouei AE. Physiotherapy for women with stress urinary incontinence: a review article. Journal of physical therapy science. 2014;26(9):1493–9.

[8] Wyman JF, Harkins SW, Fantl JA. Psychosocial impact of urinary incontinence in the community-dwelling population. Journal of the American Geriatrics Society. 1990;38(3):282–8.

[9] Johnson TM, Kincade JE, Bernard SL, Busby-Whitehead J, Hertz-Picciotto I, DeFriese GH. The association of urinary incontinence with poor self-rated health. Journal of the American Geriatrics Society. 1998;46(6):693–9.

[10] Temml C, Haidinger G, Schmidbauer J, Schatzl G, Madersbacher S. Urinary incontinence in both sexes. Neurourol Urodyn. 2000;19:259–71.

[11] Dugan E, Cohen SJ, Bland DR, Preisser JS, Davis CC, Suggs PK, et al. The association of depressive symptoms and urinary incontinence among older adults. Journal of the American Geriatrics Society. 2000;48(4):413–6.

[12] Hermansen IL, O'Connell BO, Gaskin CJ. Women's explanations for urinary incontinence, their management strategies, and their quality of life during the postpartum period. Journal of Wound Ostomy & Continence Nursing. 2010;37(2):187–92.

[13] Thüroff JW, Abrams P, Andersson K-E, Artibani W, Chapple CR, Drake MJ, et al. EAU guidelines on urinary incontinence. Actas Urológicas Españolas (English Edition). 2011;35(7):373–88.

[14] Abrams P, Cardozo L, Khoury S, Wein AJ. Incontinence: 5th International Consultation on Incontinence, Paris, February 2012: ICUD-EAU; 2013.

[15] Abbas TR, Ibrahim MA, Abogamal AF. Conservative management of stress urinary incontinence by biofeedback-assisted pelvic floor physiotherapy. Med. J. Cairo Univ. 2012;80(1):785–792.

[16] Shamliyan T, Wyman J, Kane RL. Nonsurgical Treatments for Urinary Incontinence in Adult Women: Diagnosis and Comparative Effectiveness. Rockville (MD): Agency for Healthcare Research and Quality (US); 2012 Apr. (Comparative Effectiveness Reviews, No. 36). [updated 23.12.2016; cited 03.05.2016]. Available from: https://www.ncbi.nlm.nih.gov/books/NBK92960/

[17] Nygaard IE, Heit M. Stress urinary incontinence. Obstetrics & Gynecology. 2004;104(3):607–20.

[18] Lo SK, Naidu J, Cao Y. Additive effect of interferential therapy over pelvic floor exercise alone in the treatment of female urinary stress and urge incontinence: a randomized controlled trial. Hong Kong Physiotherapy Journal. 2003;21(1):37–42.

[19] Nishizawa O, Ishizuka O, Okamura K, Gotoh M, Hasegawa T, Hirao Y. Guidelines for management of urinary incontinence. International Journal of Urology. 2008;15(10):857–74.

[20] Castro R, Arruda R, Bortolini M. Female urinary incontinence: effective treatment strategies. Climacteric. 2015;18(2):135–41.

[21] Kristen Cook LMS. Urinary Incontinence in the Older Adult. Pharmacotherapy Self-Assessment Program (PSAP). Special Populations. 2013. [updated 23.12.2016; cited 01.05.2016]. Available from: https://www.accp.com/docs/bookstore/psap/p13b2_m1ch.pdf

[22] Shamliyan T, Wyman J, Bliss DZ, Kane RL, Wilt TJ. Prevention of urinary and fecal incontinence in adults. Evidence Report/Technology Assessment. 2007(161):1–379.

[23] National Institute for Clinical Excellence, NICE: Urinary incontinence: the management of urinary incontinence in women. Clinical Guideline. October 2006.

[24] Akkus Y, Pinar G. Evaluation of the prevalence, type, severity, and risk factors of urinary incontinence and its impact on quality of life among women in Turkey. International Urogynecology Journal. 2015:1–7.

[25] Faiena I, Patel N, Parihar JS, Calabrese M, Tunuguntla H. Conservative management of urinary incontinence in women. Reviews in Urology. 2015;17(3):129.

[26] Abrams P, Cardozo L, Fall M, Griffiths D, Rosier P, Ulmsten U, et al. The standardisation of terminology of lower urinary tract function: report from the Standardisation Sub-committee of the International Continence Society. American Journal of Obstetrics and Gynecology. 2002;187(1):116–26.

[27] Haylen BT, Freeman RM, Swift SE, Cosson M, Davila GW, Deprest J, et al. An International Urogynecological Association (IUGA)/International Continence Society (ICS) joint terminology and classification of the complications related directly to the insertion of prostheses (meshes, implants, tapes) and grafts in female pelvic floor surgery. Neurourology and Urodynamics. 2011;30(1):2–12.

[28] Bettez M, Le Mai Tu KC, Corcos J, Gajewski J, Jolivet M, Bailly G. 2012 update: guidelines for adult urinary incontinence collaborative consensus document for the Canadian Urological Association. Canadian Urological Association Journal. 2012;6(5):354.

[29] Lim R, Lee SWH, Tan PY, Liong ML, Yuen KH. Efficacy of electromagnetic therapy for urinary incontinence: a systematic review. Neurourology and Urodynamics. 2015;34(8):713–22.

[30] Parsons M, Cardozo L. The classification of urinary incontinence. Reviews in Gynaecological Practice. 2003;3(2):57–64.

[31] Schreiner L, Santos TGd, Souza ABAd, Nygaard CC. Electrical stimulation for urinary incontinence in women: a systematic review. International Brazilian Journal of Urology. 2013;39(4):454–64.

[32] Rai J, Parkinson R. Urinary incontinence in adults. Surgery (Oxford). 2014;32(6):286–91.

[33] Hassan AS, Hassan O. Interfential therapy vs. pelvic floor exercises for the treatment of stress urinary incontinence in women. Egyptian Rheumatology and Rehabilitation.2003;30(1)

[34] Burgio KL. Update on behavioral and physical therapies for incontinence and overactive bladder: the role of pelvic floor muscle training. Current Urology Reports. 2013;14(5):457–64.

[35] Shamliyan TA, Kane RL, Wyman J, Wilt TJ. Systematic review: randomized, controlled trials of nonsurgical treatments for urinary incontinence in women. Annals of Internal Medicine. 2008;148(6):459–73.

[36] Mantle J. Physiotherapy for incontinence.In:Cardozo L, Staskin D eds.Textbook of female urology and urogynaecology.London:Isis Medical Media.2001;351–358.

[37] Price N, Dawood R, Jackson SR. Pelvic floor exercise for urinary incontinence: a systematic literature review. Maturitas. 2010;67(4):309–15.

[38] Dumoulin C, Hay-Smith J, Mac Habee-Seguin G. Pelvic floor muscle training versus no treatment, or inactive control treatments, for urinary incontinence in women. Cochrane Database of Systematic Review. 2014;5,14.

[39] Ayeleke RO, Hay-Smith EJC, Omar MI. Pelvic floor muscle training added to another active treatment versus the same active treatment alone for urinary incontinence in women. Cochrane Database of Systematic Reviews 2015;11,7.

[40] DeLancey JO. Structural support of the urethra as it relates to stress urinary incontinence: the hammock hypothesis. American Journal of Obstetrics and Gynecology. 1994;170(6):1713–23.

[41] Richmond CF, Martin DK, Yip SO, Dick MA, Erekson EA. Effect of supervised pelvic floor biofeedback and electrical stimulation in women with mixed and stress urinary incontinence. Female Pelvic Medicine & Reconstructive Surgery. 2016;22(5):324–7.

[42] Peschers U, Gingelmaier A, Jundt K, Leib B, Dimpfl T. Evaluation of pelvic floor muscle strength using four different techniques. International Urogynecology Journal. 2001;12(1):27–30.

[43] Haslem J. Therapeutic management of incontinence and pelvic pain. Springer, London. 2007.

[44] Bø K, Hilde G. Does it work in the long term?—A systematic review on pelvic floor muscle training for female stress urinary incontinence. Neurourology and Urodynamics. 2013;32(3):215–23.

[45] Luginbuehl H, Lehmann C, Baeyens J-P, Kuhn A, Radlinger L. Involuntary reflexive pelvic floor muscle training in addition to standard training versus standard training alone for women with stress urinary incontinence: study protocol for a randomized controlled trial. Trials. 2015;16(1):524.

[46] Enhorning G. Simultaneous recording of intravesical and intra-urethral pressure. A study on urethral closure in normal and stress incontinent women. Acta Chirurgica Scandinavica Supplementum. 1961;276:1–68.

[47] Kegel AH. Progressive resistance exercise in the functional restoration of the perineal muscles. American Journal of Obstetrics & Gynecology. 1948;56(2):238–48.

[48] Dumoulin C, Glazener C, Jenkinson D. Determining the optimal pelvic floor muscle training regimen for women with stress urinary incontinence. Neurourology and Urodynamics. 2011;30(5):746–53.

[49] Kammerer-Doak D, Rizk DE, Sorinola O, Agur W, Ismail S, Bazi T. Mixed urinary incontinence: international urogynecological association research and development committee opinion. International Urogynecology Journal. 2014;25(10):1303–12.

[50] Lamin E, Parrillo LM, Newman DK, Smith AL. Pelvic floor muscle training: underutilization in the USA. Current Urology Reports. 2016;17(2):1–7.

[51] Bø K. Pelvic floor muscle training is effective in treatment of female stress urinary incontinence, but how does it work? International Urogynecology Journal. 2004;15(2):76–84.

[52] Keane DP, O'Sullivan S. Urinary incontinence: anatomy, physiology and pathophysiology. Best Practice & Research Clinical Obstetrics & Gynaecology. 2000;14(2):207–26.

[53] Newman DK, Wein AJ. Office-based behavioral therapy for management of incontinence and other pelvic disorders. Urologic Clinics of North America. 2013;40(4):613–35.

[54] Siegel AL. Pelvic floor muscle training in males: practical applications. Urology. 2014;84(1):1–7.

[55] Miller JM, Ashton-Miller JA, DeLancey JO. A pelvic muscle precontraction can reduce cough-related urine loss in selected women with mild SUI. Journal of the American Geriatrics Society. 1998;46(7):870–4.

[56] Sangsawang B, Sangsawang N. Is a 6-week supervised pelvic floor muscle exercise program effective in preventing stress urinary incontinence in late pregnancy in primigravid women? A randomized controlled trial. European Journal of Obstetrics & Gynecology and Reproductive Biology. 2016;197:103–10.

[57] Gynecologists ACoOa. Urinary incontinence in women. Obstetrics and Gynecology. 2005(105):1533–45.

[58] Heather Stearman RB, Leilani St Anna,. How can we effectively treat stress urinary incontinence without drugs or surgery? The Journal of Family Practice. 2014;63(4).

[59] Abrams P, Andersson K, Birder L, Brubaker L, Cardozo L, Chapple C, et al. Fourth International Consultation on Incontinence Recommendations of the International Scientific Committee: evaluation and treatment of urinary incontinence, pelvic organ prolapse, and fecal incontinence. Neurourology and Urodynamics. 2010;29(1):213–40.

[60] Bø K. Pelvic floor muscle training in treatment of female stress urinary incontinence, pelvic organ prolapse and sexual dysfunction. World Journal of Urology. 2012;30(4):437–43.

[61] Bernards ATM BL, van Heeswijk-Faase IC, et al. KNGF Guideline for physical therapy in patients with stress urinary incontinence. de Fysiotherapeut Royal Dutch Society for Physical Therapy. 2011;121:1–43.

[62] Yamanishi T, Yasuda K, Sakakibara R, Hattori T, Ito H, Murakami S. Pelvic floor electrical stimulation in the treatment of stress incontinence: an investigational study and a placebo controlled double-blind trial. The Journal of Urology. 1997;158(6):2127–31.

[63] Magali Robert SR. Conservative management of urinary incontinence,SOGC Clinical Practice Guideline. Journal of Obstetrics and Gynaecology Canada. 2006;28(12):1113–8.

[64] Borello-France D, Burgio KL. Nonsurgical treatment of urinary incontinence. Clinical Obstetrics and Gynecology. 2004;47(1):70–82.

[65] Yamanishi T, Kamai T, Yoshida KI. Neuromodulation for the treatment of urinary incontinence. International Journal of Urology. 2008;15(8):665–72.

[66] Siddiqui NY, Wu JM, Amundsen CL. Efficacy and adverse events of sacral nerve stimulation for overactive bladder: a systematic review. Neurourology and Urodynamics. 2010;29(S1):S18–S23.

[67] Ruiz BC, Outeiriño XP, Martí PC, Dueñas EL, López AL. Peripheral afferent nerve stimulation for treatment of lower urinary tract irritative symptoms. European Urology. 2004;45(1):65–9.

[68] Bower W, Moore K, Adams R, Shepherd R. A urodynamic study of surface neuromodulation versus sham in detrusor instability and sensory urgency. The Journal of Urology. 1998;160(6):2133–6.

[69] Berghmans L, Hendriks H, De Bie R, Van Waalwijk E, Doorn V, Bø K, et al. Conservative treatment of urge urinary incontinence in women: a systematic review of randomized clinical trials. BJU International. 2000;85(3):254–63.

[70] Stewart F, Gameiro OL, El Dib R, Gameiro MO, Kapoor A, Amaro JL. Electrical stimulation with non-implanted electrodes for overactive bladder in adults. Cochrane Database of Systematic Reviews 2016;(12).

[71] Messelink E. The overactive bladder and the role of the pelvic floor muscles. BJU International. 1999;83(S2):31–5.

[72] Chêne G, Mansoor A, Jacquetin B, Mellier G, Douvier S, Sergent F, et al. Female urinary incontinence and intravaginal electrical stimulation: an observational prospective study. European Journal of Obstetrics & Gynecology and Reproductive Biology. 2013;170(1):275–80.

[73] Apostolidis A. Neuromodulation for intractable OAB. Neurourology and Urodynamics. 2011;30(5):766–70.

[74] Wilson, P.D., Bo, K., Hay-Smith, J., Nygaard, I., Staskin, D., Wyman, J., Bourcier, A. Conservative treatment in women. Incontinence. Health Publication Ltd., Plymouth, UK; 2002:571–624.

[75] Bernards AT, Berghmans BC, Slieker-ten Hove MCP, Staal JB, de Bie RA, Hendriks EJ. Dutch guidelines for physiotherapy in patients with stress urinary incontinence: an update. International Urogynecology Journal. 2014;25(2):171–9.

[76] Brubaker L. Electrical stimulation in overactive bladder. Urology. 2000;55(5):17–23.

[77] Smith A, Hosker G, Warrell D. The role of pudendal nerve damage in the aetiology of genuine stress incontinence in women. BJOG: An International Journal of Obstetrics & Gynaecology. 1989;96(1):29–32.

[78] Eriksen B, Eik-Nes S. Long-term electrostimulation of the pelvic floor: primary therapy in female stress incontinence? Urologia Internationalis. 1989;44(2):90–5.

[79] Oláh KS, Bridges N, Denning J, Farrar DJ. The conservative management of patients with symptoms of stress incontinence: a randomized, prospective study comparing weighted vaginal cones and interferential therapy. American Journal of Obstetrics and Gynecology. 1990;162(1):87–92.

[80] Bo K. Physiotherapy to treat genuine stress incontinence. Int Cont Surv. 1996;6(2),2–3.

[81] Berghmans LCM. Conservative treatment for women with stress incontinence and bladder overactivity: Maastricht: Maastricht University.2000; 127.

[82] Bø K. Is there still a place for physiotherapy in the treatment of female incontinence? EAU Update Series. 2003;1(3):145–53.

[83] Fall M, Lindström S. Electrical stimulation. A physiologic approach to the treatment of urinary incontinence. The Urologic Clinics of North America. 1991;18(2):393–407.

[84] Scheepens W, Van Koeveringe G, De Bie R, Weil E, van Kerrebroeck PE. Urodynamic results of sacral neuromodulation correlate with subjective improvement in patients with an overactive bladder. European Urology. 2003;43(3):282–7.

[85] Weil E, Ruiz-Cerda J, Eerdmans P, Janknegt R, Bemelmans B, van Kerrebroeck PE. Sacral root neuromodulation in the treatment of refractory urinary urge incontinence: a prospective randomized clinical trial. European Urology. 2000;37(2):161–71.

[86] Sandweiss JH. Biofeedback and sports science. New York. Springer; 1985.

[87] Herderschee R, Hay-Smith EJC, Herbison GP, Roovers JP, Heineman MJ. Feedback or biofeedback to augment pelvic floor muscle training for urinary incontinence in women. Cochrane Database of Systematic Review. 2011;7,4.

[88] Pages I-H, Jahr S, Schaufele MK, Conradi E. Comparative analysis of biofeedback and physical therapy for treatment of urinary stress incontinence in women. American Journal of Physical Medicine & Rehabilitation. 2001;80(7):494–502.

[89] Wang S, Lv J, Feng X, Wang G, Lv T. Efficacy of electrical pudendal nerve stimulation in treating female stress incontinence. Urology. 2016;91:64–9.

[90] Kielb SJ. Stress incontinence: alternatives to surgery. International Journal of Fertility and Women's Medicine. 2004;50(1):24–9.

[91] Smith AL, Moy ML. Modern management of women with stress urinary incontinence. Ostomy/wound Management. 2004;50(12):32–9; quiz 40–1.

[92] Yamanishi T, Yasuda K. Electrical stimulation for stress incontinence. International Urogynecology Journal. 1998;9(5):281–90.

[93] Hay-Smith J, Bo K, Berghmans B, Hendriks E, de Bie R, van Waalwijk van Doorn E. Pelvic floor muscle training for urinary incontinence in women. New Zealand.The Cochrane Library. 2001.

[94] Neumann PB, Grimmer KA, Deenadayalan Y. Pelvic floor muscle training and adjunctive therapies for the treatment of stress urinary incontinence in women: a systematic review. BMC Women's Health. 2006;6(1):1.

[95] Moore K, Dumoulin C, Bradley C, Burgio K, Chambers T, Hagen S, et al. Adult conservative management. Abrams P, Cardozo L Khouy S, Wein A (eds): Incontinence 5th edn Committee. 2013;12:1101–227.

[96] Herbison GP, Dean N. Weighted vaginal cones for urinary incontinence. Cochrane Database of Systematic Review. 2013;7,3.

[97] Bump RC, Hurt WG, Fantl JA, Wyman JF. Assessment of Kegel pelvic muscle exercise performance after brief verbal instruction. American Journal of Obstetrics and Gynecology. 1991;165(2):322–9.

[98] Plevnik S. New method for testing and strengthening of pelvic floor muscles. Proceedings of the 15th Annual Meeting of the International Continence Society, London. 1985:267–8.

[99] Herbison P, Plevnik S, Mantle J. Weighted vaginal cones for urinary incontinence. Cochrane Database of Systematic Review. 2002;1,3.

[100] Deindl F, Schüssler B, Vodusek D, Hesse U. Neurophysiologic effect of vaginal cone application in continent and urinary stress incontinent women. International Urogynecology Journal. 1995;6(4):204–8.

[101] Wise B, Haken J, Cardozo L, Plevnik S. A comparative study of vaginal cone therapy, cones+ Kegel exercises, and maximal electrical stimulation in the treatment of female genuine stress incontinence. Neurourology and Urodynamics. 1993;12:76.

[102] Peattie A, Plevnik S, Stanton S. Vaginal cones: a conservative method of treating genuine stress incontinence. BJOG: An International Journal of Obstetrics & Gynaecology. 1988;95(10):1049–53.

[103] Gormley EA, Lightner DJ, Burgio KL, Chai TC, Clemens JQ, Culkin DJ, et al. Diagnosis and treatment of overactive bladder (non-neurogenic) in adults: AUA/SUFU guideline. The Journal of Urology. 2012;188(6):2455–63.

[104] Yüce T, Dökmeci F, Çetinkaya SE. A prospective randomized trial comparing the use of tolterodine or weighted vaginal cones in women with overactive bladder syndrome. European Journal of Obstetrics & Gynecology and Reproductive Biology. 2016;197:91–7.

[105] Foster RT, Barber MD, Parasio MFR, Walters MD, Weidner AC, Amundsen CL. A prospective assessment of overactive bladder symptoms in a cohort of elderly women who underwent transvaginal surgery for advanced pelvic organ prolapse. American Journal of Obstetrics and Gynecology. 2007;197(1):82. e1–e4.

[106] Lipp A, Shaw C, Glavind K. Mechanical devices for urinary incontinence in women. Cochrane Database of Systematic Review. 2014;12.

[107] Staskin D, Bavendam T, Miller J, Davila GW, Diokno A, Knapp P, et al. Effectiveness of a urinary control insert in the management of stress urinary incontinence: early results of a multicenter study. Urology. 1996;47(5):629–36.

[108] Galloway NT, El-Galley RE, Sand PK, Appell RA, Russell HW, Carlan SJ. Extracorporeal magnetic innervation therapy for stress urinary incontinence. Urology. 1999;53(6):1108–11.

[109] Quek P. A critical review on magnetic stimulation: what is its role in the management of pelvic floor disorders? Current Opinion in Urology. 2005;15(4):231–5.

[110] Goldberg RP, Sand PK. Electromagnetic pelvic floor stimulation: applications for the gynecologist. Obstetrical & Gynecological Survey. 2000;55(11):715–20.

[111] Ismail S, Forward G, Bastin L, Wareham K, Emery S, Lucas M. Extracorporeal magnetic energy stimulation of pelvic floor muscles for urodynamic stress incontinence of urine in women. Journal of Obstetrics and Gynaecology. 2009;29(1):35–9.

[112] Fujishiro T, Takahashi S, Enomoto H, Ugawa Y, Ueno S, Kitamura T. Magnetic stimulation of the sacral roots for the treatment of urinary frequency and urge incontinence: an investigational study and placebo controlled trial. The Journal of Urology. 2002;168(3):1036–9.

[113] Yamanishi T, Homma Y, Nishizawa O, Yasuda K, Yokoyama O. Multicenter, randomized, sham-controlled study on the efficacy of magnetic stimulation for women with urgency urinary incontinence. International Journal of Urology. 2014;21(4):395–400.

Chapter 5

Medical and Surgical Treatment for Overactive Bladder

Rodrigo Garcia-Baquero, Madurga Patuel Blanca,
Lafuente Molinero Candelaria and
Alvarez-Ossorio Jose Luis

Additional information is available at the end of the chapter

http://dx.doi.org/10.5772/66709

Abstract

In this chapter, we focus on the medical treatment of overactive bladder (OAB) syndrome. The treatment of choice of the OAB syndrome is still the anticholinergic therapy, although we must consider β3-agonists with almost the same evidence. No drug has been shown to be clearly superior to the rest. The use of oxybutynin transdermal should be considered when the side effects due to the oral administration are intolerable. In elderly patients, first efforts should be directed to use non-drug therapies, such as behavioural therapy. In patients suffering from cognitive dysfunctions, the use of antimuscarinic with caution is recommended. Mirabegron, a β3-agonist, can be offered, although it should be noted that the long-term effects are still unknown. The logical second-line treatment is the intravesical injection of botulinum toxin A, considering its temporary effectiveness and the possibility of retention. In some centres, sacral nerve stimulation may be an option. Surgical treatment should be reserved when conservative therapies fail.

Keywords: medical treatment, overactive bladder, antimuscarinics

1. Introduction

Overactive bladder or detrusor overactivity is characterized by the presence of involuntary detrusor contractions that may be spontaneous or provoked [1]. Clinically, idiopathic detrusor overactivity is manifested as the urgent desire to urinate, with or without incontinence, generally associated with frequency and nocturia, which severely affect patients' quality of life. This combination of symptoms is included in a more general term that we know of as overactive bladder (OAB) [2].

When designing a treatment algorithm, the balance between the risks and benefits of each option must be taken into account regarding effectiveness and invasiveness, and the duration, severity and reversibility of adverse effects, more so than the evidence available. Behavioural treatment or hygienic-dietetic measures, that is, pelvic floor rehabilitation exercises and bladder training, are considered to be the first line of treatment for OAB syndrome, although they require great amount of time and effort from both the physician and the patient [3]. Oral and transdermal drugs are the second line of treatment, where antimuscarinic agents, in spite of their effectiveness, present a high percentage of side effects (all reversible). The third line of treatment includes intra-bladder treatment with onabotulinum toxin A, which entails risks of urinary retention with delayed resolution, and the different options of neuromodulation and nerve stimulation, which are more invasive and require greater motivation on behalf of the patient. And finally, surgery, the last therapeutic option due to its irreversible side effects [4] is surgery such as augmentation enterocystoplasty or urinary derivation.

The medical treatment of idiopathic OAB syndrome is the main objective in this chapter.

2. Oral medication

Medical treatment is the second line of treatment of OAB syndrome. It should be highlighted that the efficacy of said treatment is subject to the associated side effects of the drugs implemented, which are usually frequent and intense, leading many patients to abandon treatment.

In an attempt to inhibit the contractions of the detrusor muscle that occur in OAB syndrome, different drugs have been used including anticholinergics, calcium antagonists (nifedipine, flunarizine and terodiline hydrochloride), β-adrenergic agonists (clenbuterol), α-adrenergic blockers (prazosin), prostaglandin-synthetase inhibitors (indomethacin) and muscle relaxants (flavoxate hydrochloride and dicyclomine) [5]. Of all the aforementioned, the most frequently used are the antimuscarinic anticholinergic drugs. Recently, a new group of drugs has become available, known as β3-agonists, which present a competitive efficacy and tolerability when compared with the classical treatment.

2.1. Antimuscarinic drugs

Antimuscarinic or anticholinergic drugs are currently used as the primary treatment of OAB syndrome. The differences among them are based on their pharmacological profiles (muscarinic receptor affinity and other routes of action), the pharmacokinetic properties (liposolubility) and the formulations available.

Antimuscarinic drugs act by blocking the muscarinic receptors that are stimulated by acetylcholine, which is simultaneously released by the parasympathetic nervous system's activity, inhibiting the contraction of the detrusor muscle. The muscarinic receptors are primarily found in smooth muscle fibres, including the detrusor muscle, and in glands. Five types of muscarinic receptors have been described in human bladders; the most frequent are M2 and

M3, with M2 predominant to M3 in a 3:1 ratio. The M2 receptors are responsible for relaxing the detrusor muscle. The M3 receptors control the contraction of the detrusor muscle. Close to 90% of the muscarinic receptors in the salivary glands are of the M3 type [6]. The concomitant stimulation of these receptors by the antimuscarinics explains the well-known adverse effects of dry mouth and constipation.

The antimuscarinics can be divided into the following groups:

- Tertiary amines (atropine, oxybutynin, propiverine, darifenacin, tolterodine and solifenacin), which are well absorbed in the gastrointestinal tract, and depending on their lipophilic nature, they present a greater or lesser capacity to pass through the blood-brain barrier.
- Quaternary amines (propantheline, trospium chloride), which are not well absorbed in the digestive tract but have a lower incidence of side effects affecting the central nervous system.

Antimuscarinic drugs are metabolized by the cytochrome P450 enzyme system, fundamentally by the CYP2D6 and CYP3A4 enzymes, with the respective risk of pharmacological interaction by enzymatic induction or inhibition.

Establishing solid criteria regarding the resolution or improvement of urinary urgency associated with OAB is difficult. The absence of a standard definition of improvement or worsening impedes the possibility of creating a concept of resolution as a primary objective. Generally, systematic reviews assert that the effect of pharmacological treatment is weak but significantly superior than that of the placebo.

Antimuscarinics lack complete selectivity at the bladder level and produce side effects in other organs and systems that may limit their use [7]. Dryness of the mouth is the most frequent side effect, although constipation, blurry vision, tachycardia, fatigue or altered cognitive function may also occur. These side effects are dose-dependent and thus patients should start with a minimal dose and gradually increase depending on the efficacy and the patient's tolerance.

The immediate release (IR) formulation of oxybutynin is the prototype drug for urinary urgency. It provides adequate flexibility regarding the maximum dose, even when used as needed 'off label'. However, due to its pharmacokinetic properties, the IR drugs have a greater risk of side effects than the extended release (ER) versions. The transdermal release system or topical gels provide an alternative formulation to be taken into consideration.

2.2. Dosage: pharmacokinetics

The dosage and pharmacokinetics of the primary antimuscarinics used in daily clinical practice are presented in **Table 1**.

All antimuscarinics are contraindicated in patients with closed-angle glaucoma. On the other hand, the use of any antimuscarinic must be taken into account during breastfeeding as it may inhibit the production of milk due to its direct effect on the mammary glands.

	Dosage	Half life	Bioavailability	Stable concentration time	Excreted in urine	Excreted in faeces	Other
Oral oxybutynin*1	IR—5 mg/8–12 h ER—10 mg/24 h	2–3 h	2–11%	8 days	50%	50%	–
Transdermal oxybutynin*2	36 mh/3–4 days (patch)	2–3 h	–	48 h	<0.1%	99%	No first hepatic pass
Tolterodine*3	IR—2 mg/1–2 h ER—4 mg/24 h	6–10 h	17–65%	4 days	77%	17%	–
Solifenacin*4	5 mg/2–4 h (max 10 mg)	50 h	90%	24 h	70%	23%	–
Fesoterodine*7	4 mg/24 h (max 8 mg)	7 h	52%	24 h	70%	7%	No first hepatic pass

*1 **Oral oxybutynin.** Oxybutynin has been the most used drug for many years to treat OAB. Along with its anticholinergic effect, it acts as an antispasmodic agent, muscle relaxant and even as a local anaesthetic, if using intra-bladder administration (*Oral Oxybutynin data sheet*).

*2 **Transdermal oxybutynin.** The transdermal route is one of the tested forms of administration to minimize side effects along with the rectal route [8, 9]. The transdermal administration of oxybutynin avoids gastrointestinal metabolism and the hepatic first-pass effect, which reduces the formation of the N-desethyl metabolite, whose plasmatic concentration is directly related with the incidence of side effects associated with antimuscarinics. Its side effect profile is similar to the placebo except for the incidence of cutaneous reactions. This leads to a high degree of compliance (90–95%) [10] (*Transdermal Oxybutynin data sheet*).

*3 **Tolterodine.** Tolterodine is an anticholinergic agent with greater selectivity on the bladder than on the salivary glands, due to its more selective antimuscarinic effect on the M2 receptors, although it seems that the M3 glandular receptors are more sensitive to blocking [11, 12].

The half-life of oral tolterodine is approximately 6 h in fast metabolizers, and around 10 h in slow-metabolizing patients (those lacking CYP2D6). The absolute bioavailability of tolterodine is 17% in fast metabolizers, which includes most patients, and 65% in slow-metabolizing patients (*Tolterodine data sheet*).

*4 **Solifenacin.** The in vitro and in vivo pharmacological studies indicate that solifenacin is a competitive inhibitor specific to sub-type M3 muscarinic receptors (*Solifenacin data sheet*).

*5 **Fesoterodine.** Fesoterodine is rapidly and extensively hydrolysed by unspecific plasmatic sterases, without undergoing the hepatic first-pass effect, producing 5-hydroxymethyl derivatives, which is the main active metabolite and which makes it responsible for the pharmacological action of fesoterodine (*Fesoterodine data sheet*).

Table 1. Dosage and pharmacokinetic characteristics of the primary antimuscarinic drugs.

2.3. Evidence: clinical efficacy

The efficacy of antimuscarinic drugs has been supported by five systematic reviews of different drugs compared to placebos [13–17]. Most of the studies include patients with an average age of 55–60 years, both men and women, where no results can be extrapolated based on sex. According to the evidence, and with significant consistency between the different studies, only moderate short-term improvement of symptoms is observed with the use of antimuscarinic drugs compared to placebo. See **Table 2**.

	Number of studies	N	Relative Risk (95% CI)	Number of patients needed to treat NNT for a cure (95% CI)
Oxybutynin (IR–ER)	4	992	1.7 (1.3–2.1)	9 (6–16)
Tolterodine (IR–ER)	4	3404	1.2 (1.1–1.4)	12 (8–25)
Solifenacin	5	6304	1.5 (1.4–1.6)	9 (6–17)
Fesoterodine	2	2465	1.3 (1.1–1.5)	8 (5–17)

Table 2. Summary of the cure rate of the principal clinical trials [18].

The best indicator of the relevance of the side effects is the rate of abandonment due to intolerance, although this is not reflected in routine clinical practice. All of the formulations of fesoterodine, oxybutynin, propiverone, solifenacin, tolterodine, darifenacin and trospium offer a greater rate of improvement or resolution and a greater rate of side effects (dryness of the mouth) compared to placebo (Evidence Level (EL) 1a and 1b, respectively). Likewise, transcutaneous oxybutynin has shown a significant improvement in the number of episodes of incontinency and nocturnal urination per day compared to placebo, with improvement in urinary urgency, similar to its gel formulation [13].

2.4. Comparison between antimuscarinic drugs

The comparisons between the different antimuscarinic drugs, both in effectiveness and in side effects, are important for decision making in daily practice.

Forty randomized and controlled clinical trials have been published along with five systematic reviews [13–15, 19, 20]. Almost all of them are studies supported by the pharmaceutical industry. Generally, the titration schemes of the dose are included in the protocols for the experimental group, but not for the comparison group. They are short studies (12 weeks) and the primary objective is the modification of the symptoms of OAB more than its cure or improvement in urinary urgency, generally analysed as a secondary objective. The clinical applicability of these studies in daily clinical practice is questionable as most of the studies are of low to average quality [16].

There is not enough evidence to confirm that one antimuscarinic drug is better than another to cure or improve urinary urgency (EL 1a). However, oxybutynin ER is superior to tolterodine

IR and ER (EL 1b), solifenacin is more effective than tolterodine IR (EL 1b) and fesoterodine is more effective than tolterodine ER (EL 1b), regarding improvement of urinary urgency. None of the antimuscarinic drugs have shown to improve the related quality of life better than the others (EL 1a) [16]. In general, it is accepted that if one antimuscarinic IR drug is not effective, an ER version is offered (grade of recommendation (GR A)).

The ER formulations cause less side effects than the IR formulations (EL 1b) [16, 20]. Oxybutynin IR produces more dryness of the mouth than tolterodine and trospium ER, but less than darifenacin [16, 20]. Oxybutynin ER generally produces more dryness of the mouth than tolterodine ER, although the incidence of moderate to severe dryness of the mouth is similar (EL 1a). Transdermal oxybutynin has a lower rate of dryness of the mouth than oxybutynin IR and than tolterodine ER, but a greater rate of abandonment due to cutaneous reactions (EL 1b) [16]. In fact, the use of transdermal oxybutynin is recommended when oral antimuscarinic drugs are not tolerated due to dryness of the mouth (GR A). Solifenacin of 10 mg daily has a greater rate of dryness of the mouth than tolterodine four daily [21, 22]. The same rate of abandonment is generally observed, rewgardless of the incidence of dryness of the mouth. The primary comparative studies regarding the efficacy and adherence are shown in **Table 3**.

Performing an early check-up of the efficacy and side effects after 1 month of treatment with these patients (GR A) is recommended. On the other hand, physicians should be able to manage and treat the side effects inherent to antimuscarinic drugs (**Tables 4** and **5**). Patients must be informed regarding said effects before starting treatment.

2.5. Adherence: persistence

Most studies on antimuscarinic drugs have a short follow-up period (12 weeks), considering that adherence in clinical trials is much higher than in routine practice [23].

The adherence rate at 2 years varies from 49 to 84% according to two clinical trials with fesoterodine at 8 mg [24, 25]. The principal drugs studied regarding adherence are oxybutynin and tolterodine. The abandonment rate was very high after 12 months with tolterodine, but even higher with oxybutynin (68–95%).

	Number of studies	*N*	Relative risk (95% CI)
Effectiveness			
Oxybutynin ER vs. tolterodine ER	3	947	1.11 (0.94–1.31)
Solifenacin vs. tolterodine ER	1	1177	1.2 (1.08–1.34)
Fesoterodine vs. tolterodine	2	3312	1.1 (1.04–1.16)
Abandonment due to side effects			
Solifenacin vs. tolterodine ER	3	2755	1.28 (0.86–1.91)
Fesoterodine vs. tolterodine	4	4440	1.54 (1.21–1.97)

Table 3. Comparison of the effectiveness and abandonment rate due to side effects of the principal antimuscarinic drugs [13].

Symptomatic treatment of dry mouth
• Drink small sips of water
• Suck on sugar-free hard candies or gum
• Avoid mouthwashes with alcohol
• Oral lubricants
- Anethole trithione (sialogogue)—one tablet three times per day (50% success rate)
- Bromhexine hydrochloride (sialogogue)—30 drops three times per day (60% success rate)
- Eledoisin (drops)—three drops under tongue when needed
- Artificial saliva—nebulizations when needed (94%)
- Squeezed lemon (sialogogue) —when needed

Table 4. Symptomatic treatment of dry mouth.

Symptomatic treatment of constipation
• Diet rich in fibre and liquids
• Fibre supplements
• Regular exercise
• Normal intestinal habits

Table 5. Symptomatic treatment of constipation.

The average number of days before the drug is discontinued varies from 30 to 50 days [26]. In this sense, more than half of all patients will abandon treatment with antimuscarinics within the first 3 months due to lack of effectiveness, side effects or cost (EL 2).

Several randomized and controlled clinical trials have attempted to identify factors associated with a lower adherence rate. In this sense, the low level of efficacy (41.3%), adverse effects (22.4%) and cost (18.7%) [26] is associated with a lower adherence/persistence, along with IR formulations, age (young people), unrealistic expectations about treatment, gender (male) or race (Afro-Americans and other minorities).

2.6. Cognitive effects in old age—anticholinergic load

Few studies in the elderly population with OAB are available and they present various limitations including the multi-factorial aetiology of urinary urgency at this age, the presence of co-morbidities such as cognitive deficit, the effect of concomitant medications or the high risk of suffering side effects. However, it can be confirmed that all antimuscarinic drugs are effective in elderly patients (EL 1b).

The evidence is not conclusive regarding the cognitive effects of antimuscarinic drugs [27]. Few studies specifically study the cognitive changes associated with treatment using antimuscarinics; in fact, there are no studies conducted on patients who are vulnerable to suffering cognitive deficit.

Regarding the primary antimuscarinic drugs used, the effects on the elderly population and on cognitive function are explained as follows:

- **Oxybutynin.** There is sufficient evidence to confirm that oxybutynin IR may cause or worsen cognitive deterioration, although there is no current consensus on this topic (EL 2) [28–34].
- **Tolterodine.** No differences in the efficacy or side effects have been reported regarding age [35–38], although a greater rate of abandonment has been reported in elderly patients compared with placebo [28]. On the other hand, the post hoc analysis showed a slight negative effect on cognitive function. That said, there is no evidence that tolterodine causes deterioration of cognitive function (EL 3).
- **Solifenacin.** A cluster analysis [33] has shown that treatment with solifenacin does not increase cognitive function in elderly patients. No pharmacokinetic differences have been demonstrated between the different age groups, although a greater frequency of side effects has been observed in patients over 80 years of age, without any cognitive effects identified in healthy volunteer patients [34]. In patients with moderate cognitive deterioration, over 65 years of age, there were no differences in the efficacy between the different age groups, with a lower incidence of side effects in comparison with oxybutynin IR [33, 39]. Therefore, it can be confirmed that solifenacin has not shown to cause deterioration in cognitive function in elderly patients (EL 1b).
- **Fesoterodine.** There is no evidence in the comparison of the efficacy and side effects of fesoterodine between young and elderly patients. The cluster analysis of the different clinical trials confirmed the efficacy of fesoterodine at 8 mg but not at a dose of 4 mg in patients over 75 years of age. Adherence is lower in patients over 75 years of age; however, the effect on their mental state has not been documented [24, 40, 41]. There are no differences with the placebo regarding cognitive function in younger elderly patients [42]. Therefore, fesoterodine has not shown to cause deterioration in cognitive function in elderly patients (EL 1b).

Currently, extrapolating these data to the general elderly population is a risk. Conducting prevalence studies based on the community regarding the side effects of antimuscarinics could be very helpful in the future [43]. When antimuscarinic treatment is started in elderly patients, it is recommended that their mental function be evaluated objectively and monitored (GR C) [44]. Nonetheless, there is no consensus regarding which is the best test to evaluate mental function and detect changes in cognitive function [45, 46]. On the other hand, taking into account the so-called 'anticholinergic load' (GR C) is important in older adults. Drugs with anticholinergic properties are commonly prescribed for a variety of medical illnesses [47–50]. It has been estimated that 20–50% of older people have been prescribed at least one medication with anticholinergic activity [49, 51]. This could be long-term prescribed for conditions such as asthma or to manage the side effects of medicines used to treat psychiatric disorders [51]. That is why it is important to consider the anticholinergic load before starting a treatment with anticholinergic drugs. In this aspect, the list of potentially inappropriate medications (PIMs) determined by Beers Criteria in collaboration with the American Geriatrics Society [47] should be considered. These medications cause many problems, which are costly and often preventable in older adults and lead to poor outcomes. Some anticholinergic drugs, such as first-generation antihistamines (dexchlorpheniramine, doxylamine and hydroxyzine), antiparkinson agents (benztropine and trihexyphenidyl) and antispasmodics (scopolamine and propantheline) are considered to be avoided in this population with moderated quality of evidence and strong recommendation [47], due to the wide spectrum of central effects such as the onset of dizziness, sedation, confusion, in addition to increasing delirium, causing a decline in cognitive and physical function [49–51]. In relation to urological anticholinergic drugs such as darifenacin, trospium, fesoterodin and solifenacin, these recommendations are softer, and they are usually associated to peripheral adverse effects such as chronic constipation, dry mouth, dry eyes, blurred vision and increased heart rate [50]. Nevertheless, it is very important to estimate the anticholinergic load of each patient, in order to avoid the synergistic effect of several anticholinergic drugs, related to their tolerance and their well-known side effects [47]. Furthermore, attention should also be paid when these drugs are combined with cholinesterase inhibitors, especially in elderly patients [45].

3. β3-agonist: mirabegron

Mirabegron is the first clinical β3-agonist available. The β3-adrenergic receptors are the predominant β-receptors in the smooth muscle cells of the detrusor muscle and their stimulation leads to the relaxation of said muscle.

The clinical effectiveness of mirabegron is shown in two systematic revisions [52, 53], which demonstrate that the doses of 25, 50 and 100 mg reduce episodes of incontinency, episodes of urgency and urinary frequency in 24 h compared to placebo (EL 1a), with no differences in the frequency of side effects [52]. The continence rate (dryness) for the placebo is 35–40%, compared to 43–50% with mirabegron. In all of these studies, the significant statistical difference is observed in relation with improved symptoms, and not resolution (EL 1b). The effectiveness is similar both in those patients without previous treatment and in those that previously received treatment with antimuscarinics.

The effectiveness compared with extended release tolterodine 4 mg is practically identical with a continence rate (dryness) of 43–45% (EL 1b) [54].

The adrenergic side effects are somewhat frequent, without reaching levels of clinical relevance (EL 1a). The most frequent side effects are hypertension (7.3%), symptoms of nasopharyngitis (3.4%) and lower urinary tract infections (3%) [52]. No risks have been demonstrated with the prolongation of the QTc in electrocardiograms (ECGs) [55] nor with increased intra-ocular pressure [56] observed with the dose of 100 mg. There are no significant differences in the rate of side effects depending on the different doses of mirabegron [54]. However, it is recommended that patients be informed of the possible long-term side effects, which remain unknown (GR B).

Evaluation of urodynamic parameters in patients with OAB together with obstructive symptoms of bladder voiding concludes that mirabegron (50 or 100 mg) does not negatively affect said urodynamic voiding parameters compared with the placebo [57].

Regarding adherence, at 12 months, mirabegron presents a rate similar to that of tolterodine (5.5 vs. 3.6%, respectively) (EL 1b), although the frequency of dry mouth is significantly greater in the tolterodine group [54]. There are no studies published on its use in elderly patients with OAB.

To summarize, mirabegron seems to provide a similar efficacy as that of the antimuscarinic drugs with a clearly lower rate of dry mouth and constipation. The low incidence of uncomfortable side effects for the patient may make this the drug of choice in patients who have previously suffered from dry mouth and/or constipation and/or who are currently being treated with antimuscarinics but are unable to tolerate them [4].

If symptom control is not adequate with antimuscarinic treatment or the side effects are intolerable, along with regulating the dose, changing to a different antimuscarinic may be a suitable alternative [4]. There are various observational studies on this topic, where unsatisfied patients treated with oxybutynin [58, 59] and tolterodine [58, 60, 61] showed greater effectiveness and/or greater tolerance with solifenacin [59, 60], fesoterodine [61] or darifenacin [58]. Also, these patients could also change to a β3-adrenergic receptor antagonist such as mirabegron, with an efficacy profile similar to that of the antimuscarinic drugs but with less side effects.

The combination therapy with mirabegron and solifenacin has been evaluated previously [62]. Through a randomized, double-blind, dose-ranging, phase 2 study (called 'SYMPHONY'), it was observed that different combination therapies, mirabegron 25 and 50 mg and solifenacin 2.5, 5 and 10 mg, show significant improvements over monotherapy, solifenacin 5 mg, in relation to the mean volume voided, number of micturitions per 24 h, incontinence episodes per 24 h and urgency episodes per 24 h. All treatments were well tolerated and concordant with the known safety profile of mirabegron and solifenacin monotherapy. No dose-related trends in blood pressure, pulse rate, post-void residual volume or laboratory or ECG parameters were observed between groups, although the incidence of constipation was slightly increased with combination therapy. The lack of supra-additive effects on safety parameters demonstrated that the mild pharmacokinetic interaction between mirabegron and solifenacin that was recently described [63] did not appear to be clinically relevant. So, the combination of mirabegron and solifenacin may provide an attractive therapeutic approach to maximize efficacy and minimize the side effect burden [62].

4. Botulinum toxin

Botulinum toxin is a presynaptic neuromuscular blocker that induces a selective and reversible muscle weakness that lasts up to 6 months. Botulinum toxin exercises its paralysing effect by inhibiting the release of acetylcholine from the motor nerve to the neuromuscular junction.

http://dx.doi.org/10.5772/66709

It also decreases the afferent signals from the muscle spindles, which leads to it directly decreasing nerve activity that produces spasticity [64, 65].

The toxin marketed in Europe is onabotulinum toxin A (onabotA; BOTOX®), which is used at a dose of 100 IU dissolved in 10 ml of saline solution and injected in 20 spots on the bladder wall (0.5 ml per puncture site), over the trigone. It is indicated for the treatment of OAB with persistent or refractory urinary urgency in both sexes, in spite of the scarce number of male patients included in pre-marketing trials [66, 67]. Other doses of onabotA and other formulations of botulinum toxin A, abobotulinum toxin A and incobotulinum toxin A, have not been licensed for use in urinary urgency. Repeated injections are effective, with no decreased efficacy with repeated treatment (LE 3), but the percentage of patients who abandon treatment is high (EL 2). The most important side effects include episodes of lower urinary tract infection and increased post-urination and post-voiding volume that may require the intermittent use of a bladder catheter [68].

By studying the effect of a staggered dose, it has been established that the ideal dose of onabotA is 100 IU. The effectiveness of onabotA was shown in two randomized (1:1) phase III trials with a total of 1105 incontinent patients with OAB whose symptoms were not previously controlled with antimuscarinic treatment. In these studies, at the beginning, the population had an average of more than five episodes of urgent urinary incontinence (UUI), around 12 urinations per day and a scarce post-voiding volume. Twelve weeks after the endoscopic injection of onabotA, the episodes of UUI were reduced by half in treated patients, and to more than two, the number of urinations per day, with a total of 22.9% of patients completely dry, compared with 6.5% of the group that received injections of saline solution (EL 1a). Also, the patients' quality of life was substantially improved in the group treated with onabotA compared to the control group (EL 1a) [69]. On the other hand, the cohort studies have demonstrated the effectiveness of the injections in the bladder wall of onabotA in elderly patients [70], although the success rate was lower and the post-voiding volume was greater (>150 ml) (EL 3).

One recent clinical trial compared the injection of 100 IU of onabotA compared with solifenacin and showed similar improvement in both groups regarding UUI after 6 months [71]. The patients who received onabotA were more inclined to resolution of the UUI (27% vs. 13%, p 0.003) (EL 1a), but with greater rates of urinary retention in the first 2 months (5% vs. 0%) and urinary tract infection (33% vs. 13%). The patients who received solifenacin were more prone to suffer dry mouth.

In summary, offering endoscopic injections in the bladder wall with onabotulinum toxin A (100 U) in patients with refractory UUI after treatment with antimuscarinics (GR A) is recommended. The patients should be informed of the limited duration of the response, the risk of urinary tract infection and the possible need for posterior self-catheterizations (GR A).

5. Sacral nerve stimulation

Nerve stimulation by means of the electrical stimulation of the sacral nerve roots is currently an accepted therapeutic alternative to treat chronic urinary dysfunction when other more conservative options have failed. The development of nerve stimulation techniques has provided a more physiologic and functional vision of functional disorders of the lower urinary tract by enabling the application of electric impulses that modify the behaviour of a specific affected neuronal system.

According to the Federal Drug Administration (FDA), the indications for sacral nerve stimulation are as follows:

- UUI, due to idiopathic, post-surgical non-obstructive hyperactivity bladder overactivity, associated with faecal incontinence or urethral overactivity.
- Voiding dysfunction, due to lack of contractility of the detrusor muscle, absence of relaxation of the pelvic floor or Fowler's syndrome.
- Frequency-urgency syndrome associated or not with pelvic pain, sensorial hyperactivity or chronic cystopathies.
- Interstitial cystitis and chronic urinary dysfunction from a neurological cause, spinal cord lesions, bladder sphincter dyssynergia and stable multiple sclerosis.

Although the mechanism of action of sacral nerve stimulation is yet to be completely established, it is known that the stimulation of the sacral nerves regulates the function of the detrusor muscle and the external urinary sphincter through the inhibition or disinhibiting of the ventral inter-neurons, modulating the sacral-pontine reflexes that control urination. This is regulated through the efferent type A-β- and A-β-somatic myelinated fibres that transmit the sensorial impulses from the metameres of the S2–S4 sacral roots [72–74].

Adequate evaluation of the patient is essential before taking into consideration the use of an implant to initiate nerve stimulation, with a basic neurourological examination and a urodynamic evaluation including a flowmetry, cystomanometry and electromyography of the surface of the perineum. This study should be performed before starting treatment, during the temporary stimulation test and after the definitive insertion of the implant.

The nerve stimulation implant is inserted in two surgical times, with the establishment of three phases in the initiation of the sacral nerve stimulation:

1. Evaluation of the sacral nerves. The percutaneous insertion is carried out with fluoroscopic control using a stimulation electrode in the sacral foramen next to the sacral nerve, normally in S3. In the past, an electrode that was connected to an external stimuli generator with a cable was used for 5–7 days. Currently, a tined electrode is used that allows for a longer test phase as it avoids mobilization of the system itself [75]. At this point, the integrity of the somatic motor and sensorial fibres of the sacral roots is evaluated. The motor response in S3 is the contraction of the pelvic floor as well as plantar flexion of the first toe of the foot. The sensitive response is a tingling sensation in the perineum and external genitals.

2. Sub-chronic phase or test phase. In this phase, the therapeutic effect of the stimulation is determined through the daily urination of the patient during the stimulation. The patients who are candidates for the second surgical time for completion of the

insertion of the pulse generator are those in which the UUI is reduced by more than 50% during the test phase [76]. It has been found that the use of the serrated electrode in the initial implant increases the number of patients who end up with the definitive implant (EL 4).

3. Definitive implant. This consists of the percutaneous insertion of an electrode with four stimulation points that is implanted over the sacrum, fixing it to the periosteum and connecting it to the impulse generator placed in a subcutaneous pocket in the superior-external quadrant of the gluteus, or in the lower abdominal region [75]. The intervention is performed under general anaesthesia using short-acting muscle relaxants to reproduce the responses obtained in the evaluation of the sacral roots. The programming is performed within the first 24 h after the surgery using a telemetric programmer and selecting the individualized electric stimulation parameters of amplitude, frequency, pulse length and polarity. Also, the patient is given a hand programmer to activate or deactivate the generator and adjust the amplitude if needed.

All of the relevant randomized studies are affected by the limitation that neither the evaluators nor the patients were blinded for the active treatment decision, as all of the patients recruited for the implant had to have responded in the test phase prior to randomization.

Three clinical trials have been published regarding sacral nerve stimulation. One of them compared the implant with a control group that continued with medical treatment and delayed the implant by 6 months. Fifty per cent of the patients who were initially implanted experienced improvement of more than 90% in their UUI after 6 months compared to 1.6% of the control group [77]. Another clinical trial produced similar results; however, the effect on quality of life, evaluated using the SF-36 questionnaire, was not conclusive, with differences between groups in only one of the eight domains [78].

Reviewing a total of 17 studies of a series of cases of patient with UUI treated in the beginnings of the use of sacral nerve stimulation [79], we obtained the following results: after a follow-up period of 1–3 years, approximately 50% of the patients experienced a reduction of more than 90% in their urinary urgency, 25% showed an improvement of 50–90% and another 25% improved in less than 50%. In studies with a follow-up period of at least 4 years, the continued effectiveness of the treatment was observed, with an improvement of more than 50% of the initial symptoms in approximately 50% of the patients and a sustained resolution of symptoms in 15% (LE 3) [80, 81]. The resolution rate of UUI was 15% [81].

The incidence of adverse effects in relation with the implant is 50% [80, 81]. The most frequent adverse effect is the presence of pain at the site where the impulse generator is implanted (15.3%) followed by newly appearing pain (9%) and the migration of the electrode (8.4%) with the respective stimulation of undesired fibres and lack of effectiveness. These effects require surgical revision in 33–41% of cases [80, 81].

We can conclude that sacral nerve stimulation is more effective than maintaining conservative treatment to cure UUI (EL 1b). If available, sacral nerve stimulation should be offered to patients with UUI refractory to conservative therapies.

6. Posterior tibial nerve stimulation

Electro-stimulation is included within the conservative therapies used to treat OAB by acting on the afferent nerves of the pelvic floor. When conducting a systematic review, two clinical trials compared the action of the electro-stimulation with oxybutynin in patients with UUI, showing a similar efficacy between the two treatments [82].

Posterior tibial nerve stimulation is performed using a neuromodulator that utilizes the peroneal nerve for afferent access to the S3 spinal cord region. The mechanism that makes the neuromodulation of the bladder-urethra reflexes possible is based on the fact that the nerve fibres of the posterior tibial region share sensitive inputs with the S3 root. Current indications include overactive bladder with or without UUI and chronic pelvic pain.

The stimulation can be done in a percutaneous manner with a thin 34 G needle inserted just below the medial malleolus of the ankle (P-PTNS), although it can also be done in a transcutaneous manner (T-PTNS). Adequate stimulation applied using the neuromodulator, regarding the frequency, intensity and length of the impulses, is demonstrated when the big toe is observed flexing or the remaining toes show extension or flexion. The normal treatment scheme consists of 12 weekly sessions of 30 min.

Regarding P-PTNS and based on two clinical trials [83, 84], the results in women with refractory OAB are consistent. The results suggest that this treatment improves UUI in women who have previously received treatment with antimuscarinics that was not effective or tolerable (EL 2b) (GR B). However, there is not enough evidence to confirm that P-PTNS cures UUI or offers a long-term solution for symptoms of OAB as the therapeutic effects dissipate when the treatment ends. On the other hand, P-PTNS does not seem to be more effective than tolterodine in women (EL 1b) [85]. In men, there is no sufficient evidence to extract conclusions about its effectiveness.

Regarding T-PTNS, a small clinical trial compared T-PTNS together with standard treatment (rehabilitation of the pelvic floor and bladder training) with standard treatment used alone in elderly women. The group that received T-PTNS showed more improvement of symptoms at the end of treatment [86]. However, the evidence on T-PTNS is limited (EL 2a).

The side effects associated with this technique are infrequent and mild. The most common include cases of a painful feeling and transitory bleeding or bruising at the puncture site [87].

In routine clinical practice, finding patients on second-line (drugs) or even third-line treatment (botulinum toxin, PTNS or sacral nerve stimulation) that have not been correctly evaluated before starting said treatment, or that have never tried previous behaviour therapies, is common. Finding patients who have had little success with pharmacological treatment or with different combined simultaneous treatments without any clear evidence on the individual efficacy of each therapy is also common. Patients must be reminded about the importance of persisting over time with a new treatment (from 4 to 8 weeks if the treatment is pharmacological and from 8 to 12 weeks for behavioural therapies) to be able to clearly evaluate the efficacy and associated side effects before trying another line of treatment [4].

7. Surgical treatments

Surgical treatment is reserved when all the non-invasive therapies have not been effective. The first option is usually the augmentation cystoplasty, where a detubularized segment of bowel is inserted into the bivalved bladder wall. The distal ileum is the bowel segment most often used but any bowel segment can be used if it has the appropriate mesenteric length [88]. There are no randomized control trials comparing bladder augmentation to other treatments for patients with OAB. Most often, bladder augmentation is used to correct neurogenic OAB or small-capacity, low-compliant, bladders caused by fibrosis, tuberculosis, radiation or chronic infection. The largest case series of bladder augmentation in a mixed population of idiopathic and neurogenic OAB included 51 women [89], where only 53% were continent and satisfied with the surgery, whereas 25% had occasional leaks and 18% continued to have disabling OAB. It seems that the results for patients with idiopathic OAB (58%) seemed to be less satisfactory than for patients with neurogenic OAB (90%). Adverse effects were common and many patients may require clean intermittent self-catheterization to obtain adequate bladder emptying.

Another option is the detrusor myectomy. This technique aims to increase bladder capacity and reduce storage pressures by incising or excising a portion of the detrusor muscle, to create a pseudodiverticulum. Two case series [90, 91], in adult patients with idiopathic and neurogenic bladder dysfunction demonstrated poor long-term results caused by fibrosis of this pseudodiverticulum. This technique is rarely used nowadays.

As the last alternative, urinary diversion remains a reconstructive option for patients who decline repeated surgery for OAB. However, there are no studies that have specifically examined this technique in the treatment of non-neurogenic OAB [88].

8. Future directions

Recently, studies have been conducted to find a biomarker for OAB to broaden the pathophysiological understanding of OAB. The biomarkers studied till today's date are the nerve growth factor [92], the corticotropin-releasing factor [93], the prostaglandins [94] and inflammatory factors such as the C-reactive protein [95]. Another approach is to use high-yield DNA array profiles to identify the expression of specific genes involved in OAB [96]; however, this approach is not directed and may offer too many non-specific candidate biomarkers.

The sensorial or bladder and urethral input markers have also been studied using various methods. It remains unknown whether an ideal sensorial test for the lower urinary tract would have a clinical impact on the evaluation and management of OAB [97–99]. A recent review highlights the importance of the interaction of the bladder urothelium, the sub-urothelium and the interstitial cells with afferent sensorial fibres [100]. The urothelium is defined as a cellular compartment for sensorial transduction with urothelial cells capable of releasing and responding to specific neurotransmitters, and communicating with the afferent nerve endings inside of the urothelium [101]. The compartments of the sub-urothelium and the detrusor muscle seem to contain pacemaker-like cells, similar to the intestinal interstitial cells of Cajal, that modulate bladder contractility, rhythmicity and overactivity [102].

Both lines of research related with the basic science and translational research, once developed, will provide a greater understanding of the pathophysiological mechanisms of OAB, which would be of great help to find new therapeutic targets for the treatment of OAB syndrome.

Author details

Rodrigo Garcia-Baquero[1,2]*, Madurga Patuel Blanca[2], Lafuente Molinero Candelaria[3] and Alvarez-Ossorio Jose Luis[3]

*Address all correspondence to: rgbaquero@hotmail.com

1 European Association of Urology (EAU), European Society for Sexual Medicine (ESSM), International Society for Sexual Medicine (ISSM), Spanish Association of Urology (AEU), Spain

2 Andrology and Reconstructive Surgery Unit, Female and Functional Unit, Urology Department, Puerta del Mar University Hospital, Cadiz, Spain

3 Urology Department, Puerta del Mar University Hospital, Cadiz, Spain

References

[1] Martínez Agulló E. Terminology for lower urinary tract function. Actas Urol Esp. 2005;29:5–7.

[2] Chapple CR, Artibani W, Cardozo LD, Castro-Diaz D, Craggs M, Haab F, Khullar V, Versi E. The role of urinary urgency and its measurement in the overactive bladder symptom syndrome: current concepts and future prospects. BJU Int. 2005;95:335–40. DOI: 10.1111/j.1464-410X.2005.05294.x

[3] Borello-France D, Burgio KL, Goode PS, Markland AD, Kenton K, Balasubramanyam A, Stoddard AM. Urinary incontinence treatment network. Adherence to behavioral interventions for urge incontinence when combined with drug therapy: adherence rates, barriers, and predictors. Phys Ther. 2010;90:1493–505. DOI:10.2522/ptj.20080387

[4] Gormley EA, Lightner DJ, Burgio KL, Chai TC, Clemens JC, Culkin DJ, Das AK, Foster HE, Scarpero HM, Tessier CD, Vasavada SP. Diagnosis and treatment of overactive bladder (non-neurogenic) In Adults: AUA/SUFU Guideline. American Urological Association Education and Research, Inc. ©2012 | Amended 2014, available online at: http://www.auanet.org/education/guidelines/overactive-bladder.cfm.

[5] Wall LL. The management of detrusor instability. Clin Obstet Gynecol. 1990;33:367–77. DOI: 10.1097/00003081-199006000-00021

[6] Sigala S, Mirabella G, Peroni A, Pezzotti G, Simeone C, Spano P, Cunico SC. Differential gene expression of cholinergic muscarinic receptor subtypes in male and female normal human urinary bladder. Urology. 2002;60:719–25. DOI: 10.1016/S0090-4295(02)01819-8

[7] Guay DR. Clinical pharmacokinetics of drugs used to treat urge incontinence. Clin Pharmacokinet. 2003;42:1243–85. DOI: 10.2165/00003088-200342140-00004

[8] Anderson RU, Mobley D, Blank B, Saltzstein D, Susset J, Brown JS. Once daily controlled versus immediate release oxybutynin chloride for urge urinary incontinence. OROS Oxybutynin Study Group. J Urol. 1999;161:1809–12. DOI: 10.1016/S0022-5347(05)68810-6

[9] Winkler HA, Sand PK. Treatment of detrusor instability with oxybutynin rectal suppositories. Int Urogynecol J Pelvic Floor Dysfunct. 1998;9:100–2. DOI: 10.1007/BF01982217

[10] Cartwright R, Cardozo L. Transdermal oxybutynin: sticking to the facts. Eur Urol. 2007;51:907–14; discussion 914. DOI: 10.1016/j.eururo.2006.11.033

[11] Hills CJ, Winter SA, Balfour JA. Tolterodine. Drugs. 1998;55:813–20; discussion 821-2. 14. DOI: 10.2165/00003495-199855060-00008

[12] Nilvebrant L, Andersson KE, Gillberg PG, Stahl M, Sparf B. Tolterodine--a new bladder-selective antimuscarinic agent. Eur J Pharmacol. 1997;327:195–207. DOI: 10.1016/S0014-2999(97)89661-6

[13] Shamliyan T, Wyman J, Kane RL. Nonsurgical Treatments for Urinary Incontinence in Adult Women: Diagnosis and Comparative Effectiveness [Internet]. Rockville (MD): Agency for Healthcare Research and Quality (US); 2012.

[14] Chapple C, Khullar V, Gabriel Z, Dooley JA. The effects of antimuscarinic treatments in overactive bladder: a systematic review and meta-analysis. Eur Urol. 2005;48:5–26. DOI: 10.1016/j.eururo.2005.02.024

[15] Chapple CR, Khullar V, Gabriel Z, Muston D, Bitoun CE, Weinstein D. The effects of antimuscarinic treatments in overactive bladder: an update of a systematic review and meta-analysis. Eur Urol. 2008;54:543–62. DOI: 10.1016/j.eururo.2008.06.047

[16] McDonagh MS, Selover D, Santa J, Thakurta S. Drug Class Review: Agents for Overactive Bladder: Final Report Update 4. Portland (OR): Oregon Health & Science University; 2009.

[17] Shamliyan TA, Kane RL, Wyman J, Wilt TJ. Systematic review: randomized, controlled trials of nonsurgical treatments for urinary incontinence in women. Ann Intern Med. 2008 18;148:459–73. DOI: 10.7326/0003-4819-148-6-200803180-00211

[18] Lucas MG, Bosch RJ, Burkhard FC, Cruz F, Madden TB, Nambiar AK, Neisius A, de Ridder DJ, Tubaro A, Turner WH, Pickard RS; European Association of Urology. EAU guidelines on assessment and nonsurgical management of urinary incontinence. Eur Urol. 2012;62:1130–42. DOI: 10.1016/j.eururo.2012.08.047

[19] Hartmann KE, McPheeters ML, Biller DH, Ward RM, McKoy JN, Jerome RN, Micucci SR, Meints L, Fisher JA, Scott TA, Slaughter JC, Blume JD. Treatment of overactive bladder in women. Evid Rep Technol Assess (Full Rep). 2009;187:1-120, v.

[20] Novara G, Galfano A, Secco S, D'Elia C, Cavalleri S, Ficarra V, Artibani W. A systematic review and meta-analysis of randomized controlled trials with antimuscarinic drugs for overactive bladder. Eur Urol. 2008;54:740–63. DOI: 10.1016/j.eururo.2008.06.080

[21] Chapple C, Van Kerrebroeck P, Tubaro A, Haag-Molkenteller C, Forst HT, Massow U, Wang J, Brodsky M. Clinical efficacy, safety, and tolerability of once-daily fesoterodine in subjects with overactive bladder. Eur Urol. 2007;52:1204–12. DOI: 10.1016/j.eururo.2007.07.009

[22] Herschorn S, Swift S, Guan Z, Carlsson M, Morrow JD, Brodsky M, Gong J. Comparison of fesoterodine and tolterodine extended release for the treatment of overactive bladder: a head-to-head placebo-controlled trial. BJU Int. 2010;105:58–66. DOI: 10.1111/j.1464-410X.2009.09086.x

[23] Veenboer PW, Bosch JL. Long-term adherence to antimuscarinic therapy in everyday practice: a systematic review. J Urol. 2014;191:1003–8. DOI: 10.1016/j.juro.2013.10.046

[24] Sand PK, Heesakkers J, Kraus SR, Carlsson M, Guan Z, Berriman S. Long-term safety, tolerability and efficacy of fesoterodine in subjects with overactive bladder symptoms stratified by age: pooled analysis of two open-label extension studies. Drugs Aging. 2012 1;29:119–31. DOI: 10.2165/11597970-000000000-00000

[25] Scarpero H, Sand PK, Kelleher CJ, Berriman S, Bavendam T, Carlsson M. Long-term safety, tolerability, and efficacy of fesoterodine treatment in men and women with overactive bladder symptoms. Curr Med Res Opin. 2011;27:921–30. DOI: 10.1185/03007995.2011.559581

[26] Sears CL, Lewis C, Noel K, Albright TS, Fischer JR. Overactive bladder medication adherence when medication is free to patients. J Urol. 2010;183:1077–81. DOI: 10.1016/j.juro.2009.11.026

[27] Tannenbaum C, Paquette A, Hilmer S, Holroyd-Leduc J, Carnahan R. A systematic review of amnestic and non-amnestic mild cognitive impairment induced by anticholinergic, antihistamine, GABAergic and opioid drugs. Drugs Aging. 2012;29:639–58. DOI: 10.2165/11633250-000000000-00000

[28] Kessler TM, Bachmann LM, Minder C, Löhrer D, Umbehr M, Schünemann HJ, Kessels AG. Adverse event assessment of antimuscarinics for treating overactive bladder: a network meta-analytic approach. PLoS One. 2011;6:e16718. DOI: 10.1371/journal.pone.0016718

[29] Kay G, Crook T, Rekeda L, Lima R, Ebinger U, Arguinzoniz M, Steel M. Differential effects of the antimuscarinic agents darifenacin and oxybutynin ER on memory in older subjects. Eur Urol. 2006;50:317–26. DOI: 10.1016/j.eururo.2006.03.057

[30] Lackner TE, Wyman JF, McCarthy TC, Monigold M, Davey C. Randomized, placebo-controlled trial of the cognitive effect, safety, and tolerability of oral extended-release oxybutynin in cognitively impaired nursing home residents with urge urinary incontinence. J Am Geriatr Soc. 2008;56:862–70. DOI: 10.1111/j.1532-5415.2008.01680.x

[31] Lackner TE, Wyman JF, McCarthy TC, Monigold M, Davey C. Efficacy of oral extended-release oxybutynin in cognitively impaired older nursing home residents with urge urinary incontinence: a randomized placebo-controlled trial. J Am Med Dir Assoc. 2011;12:639–47. DOI: 10.1016/j.jamda.2010.05.003

[32] Minassian VA, Ross S, Sumabat O, Lovatsis D, Pascali D, Al-Badr A, Alarab M, Drutz HP. Randomized trial of oxybutynin extended versus immediate release for women aged 65 and older with overactive bladder: lessons learned from conducting a trial. J Obstet Gynaecol Can. 2007;29:726–32. DOI: 10.1016/S1701-2163(16)32604-4

[33] Wagg A, Dale M, Tretter R, Stow B, Compion G. Randomised, multicentre, placebo-controlled, double-blind crossover study investigating the effect of solifenacin and oxybutynin in elderly people with mild cognitive impairment: the SENIOR study. Eur Urol. 2013;64:74–81. DOI: 10.1016/j.eururo.2013.01.002

[34] Wesnes KA, Edgar C, Tretter RN, Bolodeoku J. Exploratory pilot study assessing the risk of cognitive impairment or sedation in the elderly following single doses of solifenacin 10 mg. Expert Opin Drug Saf. 2009;8:615–26. DOI: 10.1517/14740330903260790

[35] Drutz HP, Appell RA, Gleason D, Klimberg I, Radomski S. Clinical efficacy and safety of tolterodine compared to oxybutynin and placebo in patients with overactive bladder. Int Urogynecol J Pelvic Floor Dysfunct. 1999;10:283–9. DOI: 10.1007/s001929970003

[36] Michel MC, Schneider T, Krege S, Goepel M. Does gender or age affect the efficacy and safety of tolterodine J Urol. 2002;168:1027–31. DOI: 10.1016/S0022-5347(05)64567-3

[37] Millard R, Tuttle J, Moore K, Susset J, Clarke B, Dwyer P, Davis BE. Clinical efficacy and safety of tolterodine compared to placebo in detrusor overactivity. J Urol. 1999;161:1551–5. DOI: 10.1016/S0022-5347(05)68951-3

[38] Zinner NR, Mattiasson A, Stanton SL. Efficacy, safety, and tolerability of extended-release once-daily tolterodine treatment for overactive bladder in older versus younger patients. J Am Geriatr Soc. 2002;50:799–807.DOI: 10.1046/j.1532-5415.2002.50203.x

[39] Herschorn S, Pommerville P, Stothers L, Egerdie B, Gajewski J, Carlson K, Radomski S, Drutz H, Schulz J, Barkin J, Hirshberg E, Corcos J. Tolerability of solifenacin and oxybutynin immediate release in older (>65 years) and younger (≤65 years) patients with overactive bladder: sub-analysis from a Canadian, randomized, double-blind study. Curr Med Res Opin. 2011;27:375–82. DOI: 10.1185/03007995.2010.541433

[40] DuBeau CE, Morrow JD, Kraus SR, Creanga D, Bavendam T. Efficacy and tolerability of fesoterodine versus tolterodine in older and younger subjects with overactive bladder: a post hoc, pooled analysis from two placebo-controlled trials. Neurourol Urodyn. 2012;31:1258–65. DOI: 10.1002/nau.22252

[41] Kraus SR, Ruiz-Cerdá JL, Martire D, Wang JT, Wagg AS. Efficacy and tolerability of fesoterodine in older and younger subjects with overactive bladder. Urology. 2010;76:1350–7. DOI: 10.1016/j.urology.2010.03.097

[42] Kay GG, Maruff P, Scholfield D, Malhotra B, Whelan L, Darekar A, Martire DL. Evaluation of cognitive function in healthy older subjects treated with fesoterodine. Postgrad Med. 2012;124:7–15. DOI: 10.3810/pgm.2012.05.2543

[43] Ancelin ML, Artero S, Portet F, Dupuy AM, Touchon J, Ritchie K. Non-degenerative mild cognitive impairment in elderly people and use of anticholinergic drugs: longitudinal cohort study. BMJ. 2006;332:455–9. DOI: 10.1136/bmj.38740.439664.DE

[44] Wagg A, Verdejo C, Molander U. Review of cognitive impairment with antimuscarinic agents in elderly patients with overactive bladder. Int J Clin Pract. 2010;64:1279–86. DOI: 10.1111/j.1742-1241.2010.02449.x

[45] Sink KM, Thomas J 3rd, Xu H, Craig B, Kritchevsky S, Sands LP. Dual use of bladder anticholinergics and cholinesterase inhibitors: long-term functional and cognitive outcomes. J Am Geriatr Soc. 2008;56:847–53. DOI: 10.1111/j.1532-5415.2008.01681.x

[46] Wagg A, Khullar V, Michel MC, Oelke M, Darekar A, Bitoun CE. Long-term safety, tolerability and efficacy of flexible-dose fesoterodine in elderly patients with overactive bladder: open-label extension of the SOFIA trial. Neurourol Urodyn. 2014;33:106–14. DOI: 10.1002/nau.22383

[47] American Geriatrics Society 2012 Beers Criteria Update Expert Panel. American Geriatrics Society updated Beers Criteria for potentially inappropriate medication use in older adults. J Am Geriatr Soc. 2012 Apr;60(4):616–31. DOI: 10.1111/j.1532-5415.2012.03923.x

[48] Boustani M, Campbell N, Munger S, Fox C. Impact of anticholinergics on the aging brain: a review and practical application. Aging Health 2008 4(3):311–320. DOI: 10.2217/1745509X.4.3.311

[49] Cai X, Campbell N, Khan B, Callahan C, Boustani M. Long-term anticholinergic use and the aging brain. Alzheimers Dement. 2013;9:377–85. DOI:10.1016/j.jalz.2012.02.005

[50] Ness J, Hoth A, Barnett M, Shorr R, Kaboli P. Anti-cholinergic medications in community-dwelling older veterans: prevalence of anti-cholinergic symptoms, symptom burden and adverse drug events. Am J Geriatr Pharamacother 2006; 4:42–51. DOI: 10.1016/j.amjopharm.2006.03.008

[51] Campbell N, Boustani M, Limbil T, Ott C, Fox C, Maidment I, Schubert CC, Munger S, Fick D, Miller D, Gulati R. The cognitive impact of anticholinergics: a clinical review. Clin Interv Aging. 2009;4:225–33.

[52] Chapple CR, Cardozo L, Nitti VW, Siddiqui E, Michel MC. Mirabegron in overactive bladder: a review of efficacy, safety, and tolerability. Neurourol Urodyn. 2014;33:17–30. DOI: 10.1002/nau.22505

[53] Cui Y, Zong H, Yang C, Yan H, Zhang Y. The efficacy and safety of mirabegron in treating OAB: a systematic review and meta-analysis of phase III trials. Int Urol Nephrol. 2014;46:275–84. DOI: 10.1007/s11255-013-0509-9

[54] Chapple CR, Kaplan SA, Mitcheson D, Klecka J, Cummings J, Drogendijk T, Dorrepaal C, Martin N. Randomized double-blind, active-controlled phase 3 study to assess 12-month safety and efficacy of mirabegron, a β(3)-adrenoceptor agonist, in overactive bladder. Eur Urol. 2013;63:296–305. DOI:10.1016/j.eururo.2012.10.048

[55] Malik M, van Gelderen EM, Lee JH, Kowalski DL, Yen M, Goldwater R, Mujais SK, Schaddelee MP, de Koning P, Kaibara A, Moy SS, Keirns JJ. Proarrhythmic safety of repeat doses of mirabegron in healthy subjects: a randomized, double-blind, placebo-, and active-controlled thorough QT study. Clin Pharmacol Ther. 2012;92:696–706. DOI: 10.1038/clpt.2012.181

[56] Martin N, Lewis RA, Vogel R, Novack G. Randomised, double-blind, placebo-controlled study to assess the ocular safety of mirabegron in normotensive IOP research subjects. Eur Urol. 2012 11(2):e686–e686a. DOI: 10.1016/S1569-9056(12)60683-6

[57] Nitti VW, Rosenberg S, Mitcheson DH, He W, Fakhoury A, Martin NE. Urodynamics and safety of the β3-adrenoceptor agonist mirabegron in males with lower urinary tract symptoms and bladder outlet obstruction. J Urol. 2013;190:1320–7. DOI: 10.1016/j.juro.2013.05.062

[58] Zinner N, Kobashi KC, Ebinger U, Viegas A, Egermark M, Quebe-Fehling E, Koochaki P. Darifenacin treatment for overactive bladder in patients who expressed dissatisfaction with prior extended-release antimuscarinic therapy. Int J Clin Pract. 2008;62:1664–74. DOI: 10.1111/j.1742-1241.2008.01893.x

[59] Wong C, Duggan P. Solifenacin for overactive bladder in women unsuccessfully treated with immediate release oxybutynin: a pilot study. J Obstet Gynaecol 2009;29:31–4. DOI: 10.1080/01443610802628726

[60] Zinner N, Noe L, Rasouliyan L, Marshall T, Seifeldin R. Impact of solifenacin on resource utilization, work productivity and health utility in overactive bladder patients switching from tolterodine ER. Curr Med Res Opin. 2008;24:1583–91. DOI: 10.1185/03007990802081766

[61] Wyndaele JJ, Goldfischer ER, Morrow JD, Gong J, Tseng LJ, Guan Z, Choo MS. Effects of flexible-dose fesoterodine on overactive bladder symptoms and treatment satisfaction: an open-label study. Int J Clin Pract. 2009;63:560–7. DOI: 10.1111/j.1742-1241.2009.02035.x

[62] Abrams P, Kelleher C, Staskin D, Rechberger T, Kay R, Martina R, Newgreen D, Paireddy A, van Maanen R, Ridder A. Combination treatment with mirabegron and solifenacin in patients with overactive bladder: efficacy and safety results from a randomised, double-blind, dose-ranging, phase 2 study (Symphony). Eur Urol. 2015;67:577–88. DOI: 10.1016/j.eururo.2014.02.012.

[63] Krauwinkel WJJ, Kerbusch VM, Meijer J, Tretter R, Strabach G, van Gelderen EM. Evaluation of the pharmacokinetic interaction between the b3-adrenoceptor agonist mirabegron and the muscarinic receptor antagonist solifenacin in healthy subjects. Clin Pharm Drug Dev 2013;2:255–63. DOI: 10.1002/cpdd.37.

[64] Rosales RL, Arimura K, Takenaga S, Osame M. Extrafusal and intrafusal muscle effects in experimental botulinum toxin-A injection. Muscle Nerve. 1996;19:488–96. DOI: 10.1002/(SICI)1097-4598(199604)19:4%3C488::AID-MUS9%3E3.0.CO;2-8

[65] Moreno-López B, de la Cruz RR, Pastor AM, Delgado-García JM. Effects of botulinum neurotoxin type A on abducens motoneurons in the cat: alterations of the discharge pattern. Neuroscience. 1997;81:437–55. DOI: 10.1016/S0306-4522(97)00199-1

[66] Duthie JB, Vincent M, Herbison GP, Wilson DI, Wilson D. Botulinum toxin injections for adults with overactive bladder syndrome. Cochrane Databas Syst Rev. 2011;12:CD005493. DOI: 10.1002/14651858.CD005493.pub3

[67] Mangera A, Andersson KE, Apostolidis A, Chapple C, Dasgupta P, Giannantoni A, Gravas S, Madersbacher S. Contemporary management of lower urinary tract disease with botulinum toxin A: a systematic review of botox (onabotulinumtoxinA) and dysport (abobotulinumtoxinA). Eur Urol. 2011;60:784–95. DOI: 10.1016/j.eururo.2011.07.001

[68] Chapple C, Sievert KD, MacDiarmid S, Khullar V, Radziszewski P, Nardo C, Thompson C, Zhou J, Haag-Molkenteller C. OnabotulinumtoxinA 100 U significantly improves all idiopathic overactive bladder symptoms and quality of life in patients with overactive bladder and urinary incontinence: a randomised, double-blind, placebo-controlled trial. Eur Urol. 2013;64:249–56. DOI: 10.1016/j.eururo.2013.04.001

[69] Nitti VW, Dmochowski R, Herschorn S, Sand P, Thompson C, Nardo C, Yan X, Haag-Molkenteller C; EMBARK Study Group. OnabotulinumtoxinA for the treatment of patients with overactive bladder and urinary incontinence: results of a phase 3, randomized, placebo controlled trial. J Urol. 2013;189:2186–93. DOI: 10.1016/j.juro.2012.12.022

[70] White WM, Pickens RB, Doggweiler R, Klein FA. Short-term efficacy of botulinum toxin a for refractory overactive bladder in the elderly population. J Urol. 2008;180:2522–6. DOI: 10.1016/j.juro.2008.08.030

[71] Visco AG, Brubaker L, Richter HE, Nygaard I, Paraiso MF, Menefee SA, Schaffer J, Lowder J, Khandwala S, Sirls L, Spino C, Nolen TL, Wallace D, Meikle SF; Pelvic Floor Disorders Network. Anticholinergic therapy vs. onabotulinumtoxina for urgency urinary incontinence. N Engl J Med. 2012;367(19):1803–13. DOI: 10.1056/NEJMoa1208872

[72] Chancellor MB, Chartier-Kastler EJ. Principles of sacral nerve stimulation (SNS) for the treatment of bladder and urethral sphincter dysfunctions. Neuromodulation. 2000;3:16–26. DOI: 10.1046/j.1525-1403.2000.00015.x

[73] Zermann DH, Ishigooka M, Doggweiler R, Schmidt RA. Postoperative chronic pain and bladder dysfunction: windup and neuronal plasticity--do we need a more neurological approach in pelvic surgery? J Urol. 1998;160:102–5. DOI: 10.1016/S0022-5347(01)63047-7

[74] Chartier-Kastler EJ, Ruud Bosch JL, Perrigot M, Chancellor MB, Richard F, Denys P. Long-term results of sacral nerve stimulation (S3) for the treatment of neurogenic refractory urge incontinence related to detrusor hyperreflexia. J Urol. 2000;164:1476–80. DOI: 10.1016/S0022-5347(05)67010-3

[75] Spinelli M, Mamo GA, Arduini A, Gerber M, Giardello G. Evolution of a minimally invasive procedure for sacral neuromodulation. New perspectives in sacral nerve stimulation. London: Martin Dunita Eds. 2002. p 223–8.

[76] Arlandis S, Ruiz-Cerda JL, Jimenez-Cruz F. Diagnosis and patient selection. Neuromodulation, a new therapeutic alternative for lower urinary tract disorders. Madrid: ENE Eds. 2002. p. 167–88.

[77] Schmidt RA, Jonas U, Oleson KA, Janknegt RA, Hassouna MM, Siegel SW, van Kerrebroeck PE. Sacral nerve stimulation for treatment of refractory urinary urge incontinence. Sacral Nerve Stimulation Study Group. J Urol. 1999;162:352–7. DOI: 10.1016/S0022-5347(05)68558-8

[78] Weil EH, Ruiz-Cerdá JL, Eerdmans PH, Janknegt RA, Bemelmans BL, van Kerrebroeck PE. Sacral root neuromodulation in the treatment of refractory urinary urge incontinence: a prospective randomized clinical trial. Eur Urol.2000;37:161–71. DOI: 10.1159/000020134

[79] Brazzelli M, et al. Efficacy and safety of sacral nerve stimulation for urinary urge incontinence: a systematic review. J Urol 2006;175:835–41. DOI: 10.1016/S0022-5347(05)00326-5

[80] Groen J, Blok BF, Bosch JL. Sacral neuromodulation as treatment for refractory idiopathic urge urinary incontinence: 5-year results of a longitudinal study in 60 women. J Urol. 2011;186:954–9. DOI: 10.1016/j.juro.2011.04.059

[81] Van Kerrebroeck PE, van Voskuilen AC, Heesakkers JP, Lycklama á Nijholt AA, Siegel S, Jonas U, Fowler CJ, Fall M, Gajewski JB, Hassouna MM, Cappellano F, Elhilali MM, Milam DF, Das AK, Dijkema HE, van den Hombergh U. Results of sacral neuromodulation therapy for urinary voiding dysfunction: outcomes of a prospective, worldwide clinical study. J Urol. 2007;178:2029–34. DOI: 10.1016/j.juro.2007.07.032

[82] Geoffrion R; Society of Obstetricians and Gynaecologists of Canada. Treatments for overactive bladder: focus on pharmacotherapy. J Obstet Gynaecol Can. 2012;34:1092–101. DOI: 10.1016/S1701-2163(16)35440-8

[83] Finazzi-Agrò E, Petta F, Sciobica F, Pasqualetti P, Musco S, Bove P. Percutaneous tibial nerve stimulation effects on detrusor overactivity incontinence are not due to a placebo effect: a randomized, double-blind, placebo controlled trial. J Urol. 2010;184:2001–6. DOI: 10.1016/j.juro.2010.06.113

[84] Peters KM, Macdiarmid SA, Wooldridge LS, Leong FC, Shobeiri SA, Rovner ES, Siegel SW, Tate SB, Jarnagin BK, Rosenblatt PL, Feagins BA. Randomized trial of percutaneous tibial nerve stimulation versus extended-release tolterodine: results from the overactive bladder innovative therapy trial. J Urol. 2009;182:1055–61. DOI: 10.1016/j.juro.2009.05.045

[85] Civic D, Black E. Re: Randomized trial of percutaneous tibial nerve stimulation versus sham efficacy in the treatment of overactive bladder syndrome: results from the SUmiT trial: Peters KM, Carrico DJ, Perez-Marrero RA, Khan AU, Wooldridge LS, Davis GL, MacDiarmid SA. J Urol. 2010; 183:1438–43. J Urol. 2011;185:362; author reply 362-4. DOI: 10.1016/j.juro.2010.09.030

[86] Schreiner L, dos Santos TG, Knorst MR, da Silva Filho IG. Randomized trial of transcutaneous tibial nerve stimulation to treat urge urinary incontinence in older women. Int Urogynecol J. 2010;21:1065–70. DOI: 10.1007/s00192-010-1165-6

[87] Klingler HC, Pycha A, Schmidbauer J, Marberger M. Use of peripheral neuromodulation of the S3 region for treatment of detrusor overactivity: a urodynamic-based study. Urology. 2000;56:766–71. DOI: 10.1016/S0090-4295(00)00727-5

[88] Cody JD, Nabi G, Dublin N, McClinton S, Neal DE, Pickard R, Yong SM. Urinary diversion and bladder reconstruction/replacement using intestinal segments for intractable incontinence or following cystectomy. Cochrane Database Syst Rev. 2012;15:CD003306. DOI: 10.1002/14651858.

[89] Awad SA, Al-Zahrani HM, Gajewski JB, Bourque-Kehoe AA. Long-term results and complications of augmentation ileocystoplasty for idiopathic urge incontinence in women. Br J Urol. 1998;81:569–73.DOI: 10.1097/00005392-199903000-00110.

[90] Leng WW, Blalock HJ, Fredriksson WH, English SF, McGuire EJ. Enterocystoplasty or detrusor myectomy? Comparison of indications and outcomes for bladder augmentation. J Urol. 1999;161:758–63. DOI: 10.1097/00042307-199909000-00014.

[91] Ter Meulen PH, Heesakkers JP, Janknegt RA. A study on the feasibility of vesicomyotomy in patients with motor urge incontinence. Eur Urol. 1997;32:166–9.

[92] Kuo HC, Liu HT, Chancellor MB. Can urinary nerve growth factor be a biomarker for overactive bladder? Rev Urol. 2010;12:e69–77.

[93] Klausner AP, Steers WD. Corticotropin releasing factor: a mediator of emotional influences on bladder function. J Urol. 2004;172:2570–3. DOI: 10.1097/01.ju.0000144142.26242.f3

[94] Kim JC, Park EY, Seo SI, Park YH, Hwang TK. Nerve growth factor and prostaglandins in the urine of female patients with overactive bladder. J Urol. 2006;175:1773–6; discussion 1776. DOI: 10.1016/S0022-5347(05)00992-4

[95] Chung SD, Liu HT, Lin H, Kuo HC. Elevation of serum c-reactive protein in patients with OAB and IC/BPS implies chronic inflammation in the urinary bladder. Neurourol Urodyn. 2011;30:417–20. DOI: 10.1002/nau.20938

[96] Cheung W, Bluth MJ, Johns C, Khan S, Lin YY, Bluth MH. Peripheral blood mononuclear cell gene array profiles in patients with overactive bladder. Urology. 2010;75:896–901. DOI: 10.1016/j.urology.2009.06.021

[97] Kenton K, Simmons J, FitzGerald MP, Lowenstein L, Brubaker L. Urethral and bladder current perception thresholds: normative data in women. J Urol. 2007;178:189–92. DOI: 10.1016/j.juro.2007.03.032

[98] Kenton K, Lowenstein L and Brubaker L. Tolterodine causes measurable restoration of urethral sensation in women with urge urinary incontinence. Neurourol Urodyn 2010;29:555–7. DOI: 10.1002/nau.20804

[99] Fujihara A, Ukimura O, Iwata T, Miki T. Neuroselective measure of the current perception threshold of A-delta and C-fiber afferents in the lower urinary tract. Int J Urol. 2011;18:341–9. DOI: 10.1111/j.1442-2042.2011.02749.x

[100] Kanai AJ. Afferent mechanism in the urinary tract. Handb Exp Pharmacol 2011;202:171–205. DOI: 10.1007/978-3-642-16499-6_9

[101] Birder LA. Urothelial signaling. Handb Exp Pharmacol. 2011;202:207–31. DOI: 10.1007/978-3-642-16499-6_10

[102] McCloskey KD. Interstitial cells in the urinary bladder--localization and function. Neurourol Urodyn. 2010;29:82–7. DOI: 10.1002/nau.20739